MARTHA and I

Martha and I

Life, Love, and Loss in Alzheimer's Shadow

DONALD R. FLETCHER

WIPF & STOCK · Eugene, Oregon

Wipf and Stock Publishers
199 W 8th Ave, Suite 3
Eugene, OR 97401

Martha and I
Life, Love, and Loss in Alzheimer's Shadow
By Fletcher, Donald R.
Copyright©2013 by Fletcher, Donald R.
ISBN 13: 978-1-5326-3299-0
Publication date 5/17/2017
Previously published by Tate Publishing & Enterprises, LLC, 2013

To You Caregivers,
who watch and work and wait through days and years
as this relentless disease
steals a loved person out of your life,
to each of you,
now millions in this country,
giving of yourselves when you feel
there is nothing left to give,
this book is dedicated.

Acknowledgments

This book had its beginning in a visit to our home by Kevin Riordan, columnist of *The Philadelphia Inquirer*, who then wrote a feature article that stirred up these ideas. Subsequently, Marilyn Marks, editor of *The Princeton Alumni Weekly*, invited me to write on my experience with Martha. These two empathetic journalists set in motion what is offered here.

For a book as personal as this, my family has been invaluable, sharing recollections, offering insights and comments. My regret is that, given its subject, the project was undertaken only after Martha was no longer able to help me put it together. In her place, however, our daughter Sylvia has been my constant guide and support. Even while serving the United Nations overseas, she has been at my elbow through email, counseling, correcting, encouraging; and now that she is back in this country, she has continued as my mainstay in giving the book its final form.

I also acknowledge gratefully the wise help of Roger Williams, editorial consultant in Washington, DC, a skilled professional who has become a generous friend. And acknowledgement is due to the full staff of Tate Publishing, for their counsel and participation.

I hope that many of you who read these pages may find yourselves encouraged, if you also are coping in some way with what is here described.

—Donald R. Fletcher
Lions Gate, Voorhees, NJ
January 2013

Contents

Evening

So we'll talk no more, my love,
The moon is almost down.
Few words are left; none to express
What we have shared of loveliness,
Of swallows skimming grass at dusk,
And firefly sparks among the trees,
Of organ music in a shadowy nave,
One soft light only on your face and hands
And whiteness of the keys.
In our silence, now, I hold you, warm and dear
As always—hold you here, and yet not here—
Your smile flickering on the edge of time,
As you move deeper into the not-time
And I reach you less and less. Love, it's still you,
Making the passage gently, by degrees.
I'll make it, too, sometime—we still count time—
And we will talk again; or need no words
For perfect sharing—in God's harmony.

—Donald R. Fletcher
Written in Martha's Room
Skilled Nursing, Lions Gate
June 16, 2010

1

Stockings over Slacks?

2000

From the living room, I looked down the short passageway and through the open door of our bedroom to see if Martha was ready to go out with me for dinner. She wasn't. She was trying to pull on a pair of stockings over her slacks and shoes. A cold wave washed through me; but I tried to sound natural, half-bantering, as I went to her quickly.

"That doesn't really work, does it? Anyway, you're all dressed."

She looked at me, the stockings still in her hand. For just that moment, a frightening gulf seemed to open between us. Then she smiled and put the stockings in a drawer.

"Come on," I said. "This is something special, going out to dinner by ourselves—just you and I together."

It was a late afternoon in early fall, 2000. Martha and I, her husband of almost sixty years, were comfortably established in a duplex bungalow overlooking the golf course of our central New Jersey active adult community. Despite our ages—she, seventy-eight and I, eighty-one—we were both still in excellent health.

As we headed out that evening, neither of us said anything more about the stockings incident, nor did we bring it up later on. But what had occurred continued to trouble me. Had Martha noticed what she was doing? Did she wonder about it in some later awareness? It was in the nature of our relationship and our personalities, I suppose, that neither of us talked about it. Perhaps we should have, but we didn't. I tried to think of any previous hints, anything similar that I might have missed and began to watch for further clues; but none appeared as weeks went by.

☙❧

The eclipsing shadow of Alzheimer's—did anything precede it? Was there anything that brought it on? Martha and I had moved to this community, Rossmoor, because I was invited to be pastor of its ecumenical community church. We had six good years there—Martha on the organ bench and directing the music program and I in the pulpit. She was seventy-one when we moved to Rossmoor and still masterful at the organ console.

When I told Donna, the first of our children, about how Martha had tried to pull stockings over trousers, she responded with an observation that reflected her own accomplished musicianship: "What first made me think that something was affecting Mom and causing her to lose memory and/or coordination was her organ playing. I started to see a difference in how she played. She wasn't as quick to modulate and shift from one key to another, and her pedal work wasn't as agile."

Specifically, there had been the occasion of my eightieth birthday. Most of our children and some of our grandchildren gathered; and we decided that for a fun sort of celebration we would form a family chorus. At the close of the Sunday service, we'd sing the "Lutkin Benediction", a favorite that all of us had sung under Martha's direction in a variety of settings. This time, Ron—the partner of our second son, Alan— conducted with Martha at the organ. It was January of 1999, almost two years before the stocking incident. Donna noticed that her mother's playing was not up to what it had been, never mind that Martha was then into her late seventies. For my part, being with Martha all the time, I had not detected any change; and Donna said nothing to me about it at that point.

2

The Preacher's Daughter

1927

Her feet were scuffing in the bit of sand that had drifted onto the bare wood steps. Under the warm sun, a wisp of breeze brought a sound of distant waves washing at high tide under the boardwalk. The five-year-old tipped up the floppy brim of her hat, even though that made her squint against the white clapboard house fronts that lined the street. Some people were coming—that old couple from two blocks down (she didn't know them any more than that). She waited until they were almost passing, then said, "Hello. Won't you come in? Won't you stay for dinner?"

"My dear, that's very kind of you; but I don't think your mother is expecting us."

"That doesn't matter. If you come in, she'll set the table in the dining room. She only does that for company."

"Well, we really aren't company today, and we wouldn't want to put your mother to extra trouble."

"Oh, she won't mind. You will come in, won't you?"

"No, thank you, dear. We're on our way to the boardwalk. Good-bye, now."

"All right, good-bye," the girl said with a childishly exaggerated sigh.

When the couple had moved out of earshot, the husband asked his wife, "Who is that child with those blue eyes and wide smile?"

"Oh, that's the preacher's daughter. Didn't you notice that we were passing the parsonage? That's the Bradways' little girl—Martha, I think her name is."

"She's a quaint one and really persistent. I wonder what the mother would say if she knew her charming daughter was sitting out there, inviting just anyone to come in for dinner."

∽∾

Martha Bradway was bright and outgoing, and her innovative imagination sometimes put her parents, Henry and Della, to the test, making them feel they weren't as young as they used to be. And in fact they weren't young. Martha's sister was eighteen, and her brother was twelve when she was born; so, she grew up almost as an only child of older parents.

I never knew her as she was growing up, because I was on the other side of the world. As a son of a missionary doctor, I grew up in Korea—pre-WWII Korea, that was part of the Japanese Empire. Our home was in Taegu, in the southern part of the peninsula; but I went to boarding school in the north, in Pyongyang. Returning to the United States, I entered Princeton, and it was in Princeton town that my path first crossed Martha's—but that comes later in the story.

Her father was a Methodist preacher, moving from church to church in central and southern New Jersey.

18

Henry Bradway was strict on some things—such as Sunday observance and card playing—an old-school Methodist, conservative in his customs; but he was also warm, kind, and considerate. With his youngest child, he could even be indulgent. Martha was not encouraged to engage in sports; her parents gave her gym teacher a standing instruction that she was to be excused when anything like dancing was involved. But they did go along, cautiously, with her taking part in dramatic activities, which she loved.

Della was in the kitchen, as usual, when Martha burst in one afternoon in early spring. It was broad daylight, but almost dinnertime; dinner came early in the Bradway household.

"Mother, marvelous news! I got picked! I'm going to play Anne! Mrs. Carzoff had narrowed it down to Emily and me. She took us after school, had us up on the stage reading a bunch of lines. She even brought in two other teachers, and they put their heads together and talked, while we fidgeted and hoped. Then she said I would do it, with Emily as backup. Isn't that wonderful?"

"That's very good, child. Your father will be glad to hear about it. What is the name of the play again?"

"It's *Anne of Green Gables*. It's a fun play, and this is such a neat part. Daddy read the play, or most of it."

"I know. We talked about it. Everything in it is all right."

"Of course it's all right. Mrs. Carzoff wouldn't choose a play that wasn't a good play."

19

"Well, some of these plays that people think are very good have young people smoking and using language that we wouldn't want you to use."

Martha was delighted that her parents had put their stamp on the senior class theatrical production. Now she was going to play the lead. Her cup was spilling over!

She told me about it a year or so later, after we met. I didn't see a picture of her in costume—with her hair in pigtails ending in bows; but I did see her graduation snapshot in cap and gown on the front step of the parsonage. The wide smile was there and also the round eyes—blue, if the photo had been in color. Her pose looked easy and confident. High school was over; she was ready to take on a new world in college.

3

Mom Was Almost Hysterical

1999

In February 1999, I was diagnosed with bladder cancer that was treated and presumably taken care of with relatively simple surgery. But six months later, shortly after I had retired as pastor, the cancer was back, now more advanced. At the hospital of the University of Medicine and Dentistry of New Jersey, in New Brunswick, radical surgery that included internal reconstruction was offered; and the surgeons were willing to take me as a patient in spite of my age.

Martha sat in the surgical waiting room with all three daughters—Donna, Sylvia, and Marilyn. They moved around, went outside for fresh air and some food, came back, and waited. Finally, well into the evening, the twelve-hour operation was finished. Still in his surgical gear, the associate surgeon came out to report that all had gone well.

It did not continue to go well. Intestinal adhesions developed, producing a total gastrointestinal blockage that eventually required a second surgery. For weeks, I was unable to eat or drink anything. With my body weight dwindling and strength draining away, the IV served as my lifeline.

Our daughters were very concerned about my condition, and they had to be worried about their mother as well, as she tried to be constantly with me.

"Mom, you shouldn't be driving to the hospital alone."

"Why not? I can drive all right, and that's where I need to be—with Dad, while he's as sick as he is."

"Sure, Mom, you want to be with him, and we know he's glad to have you there; but you've got to think of yourself too."

That might have been Donna, protesting. As a widow, she had to get back to the piano teaching that supported her in Palo Alto, California; but for several days she and Sylvia teamed up. Sylvia, the second of our children and still single, was living and working in Washington. Without making a point of it, she and Donna took turns caring for us, one of them staying with me while the other drove Martha to and from the hospital and stayed with her while at home. Before they had to leave to go back to work, they arranged with Tom and Alan, two of our three sons, to replace them.

Tom, next in order after Sylvia, was living in a large Victorian house in Newton, outside Boston, with his wife, Janice; and Alan, fifth in line and unmarried, shared their third-floor apartment with partner Ron. Tom and Alan drove down to take over, alternating the way Donna and Sylvia had done. With the unexpected extension of my hospital stay, the whole family pitched in. Larry, the third son and our youngest and an attorney in Baltimore, came up more than once. Donna was back twice more, becoming almost a commuter on the red-eye flight from the West Coast; and her daughter Erica, eldest of our grandchildren, stayed most of the week. Marilyn, who lived in Voorhees—an hour south of our home—and the only one of our six in New Jersey, was a constant support.

One night, about eleven o'clock, Marilyn's phone rang. Sylvia's urgent voice was at the other end. The dialogue went something like this:

"Marilyn, I know it's late, but you have to come. Mom has gotten herself upset and is almost hysterical. I can't leave her this way, but I have a meeting in Washington in the morning and I've got to go."

"All right…yes. I suppose there's no way to get her calmed down."

"Nothing I know that I haven't tried. She's sure that Dad isn't going to make it. She's fixated on that idea, so I can't leave her alone in the house this way."

In three minutes, Marilyn was getting her car out of the garage. Her husband, Dale, was concerned about her starting out at that hour of the night, but she assured him that she'd make it, and that she'd be at work in the morning—maybe late.

She accomplished all of it. Martha was calmed and reassured. Marilyn achieved that. In the morning, a Rossmoor friend offered to take Martha to the hospital, and stayed there until she was ready to come home. Sylvia made it to Washington for her meeting; and though groggy after an all-night duty, Marilyn made it to work.

My hospitalization had posed a further complication for Martha and the family, which was our move within Rossmoor. We had planned selling one house to buy another with a more favorable location, before my illness and surgery came up. Even counting in the surgery and expected two-week hospital stay, the timing for the move still seemed to work. But when the stay stretched to more than six weeks, Martha had to deal with the move for both of us. Alan remembered how the stress, added to her anxiety, "made her break down quite a bit, unable to decide where the Tupperware should go or what clothing might be given away." All our children pitched in to get the move made—they vacated the old house clean, and they made the new house homelike; they even put some pictures on the walls. That's how I found the place when, still weak and shaky, I was helped from the car after that wonderfully liberating ride from the hospital and could sink down in my favorite chair. The new, refreshing view across the golf course spread before me.

In all these weeks from late August to early October, no one had a glimpse of the Alzheimer's shadow. But it was probably there—just as probably as the stress on Martha of endless hospital visits, of anxiety, of loneliness at home, and of the upheaval of a household move was advancing the disease.

4

Your Eyes Are Like the Ocean—Dangerously

1940

Martha was a freshman at Westminster Choir College, the school on the edge of Princeton town that John Finlay Williamson founded to train accomplished church musicians. Three and a half years older, I was a graduate student at the university, living on the other side of town. It's hardly likely that we would have met, except that I had a close friend Elwyn Smith, and that he had a younger sister. Elwyn's sister, Ethel, was also an entering student at Westminster. I thought I should look her up and welcome her to Princeton, as Elwyn was beginning graduate study at Harvard. So, as it happened, Ethel was getting to know Martha and introduced me to her.

I acknowledge that it wasn't love at first sight. Martha told me afterward that she took special notice of me, but my mind must have been elsewhere. In the late fall, there was a string quartet concert at the university to which I invited Ethel, bringing along a college friend who was now in seminary, and Ethel provided a date for him—Martha Bradway. In our foursome, I did take more notice of Martha that evening, finding her very pleasant. And we were together several times in the winter and early spring as officers in a church youth group—but Cupid's arrow didn't yet find a mark in me.

It wasn't until late spring that I got around to a real date, asking Martha to go with me to the closing concert given by Westminster Choir, the college's varsity chorus, in McCarter Theater. She was a vision—her slim, almost boyish shape sheathed in a long raspberry dress; her brown curls tossing and her eyes laughing, full of light. I was fascinated. The dark hair set off her white skin; but it was her eyes that drew me. They were blue, with hints of gray and green.

At that stage, I was experimenting widely with poetry as a way to express and perhaps romanticize my feelings. And I loved the sea, as I had learned to love it in summers of my boyhood in Korea. We had a cottage at Sorai Beach, a mission resort on the west coast of what is now North Korea. There we clambered over rocks, swam off a wonderfully long and curving beach, and knocked around in our small wooden sailboat.

All this I evoked in a sonnet to Martha, a day or so after our date. Was I passionate about her? Not yet. The idea of the poem was what intrigued me, although, as I developed it, I found it ending with a rather personal, romantic expression.

> Your eyes are like the ocean after rain,
> Chastened and still, grown misty to the verge
> And dim, until the sun shine out again—
> A quiet gray, far off with sky to merge.
> But when your spirit moves within the deep,
> And passion animates, a brighter sheen

Begins to glow, like waves that curl and leap
Up to a somber sky in twisted green.
Then after storm the warming sun returns,
And deep within the ocean, rolling slow,
Casts his long shafts, until the water burns
A cool, clear, even blue far down below.
Sometimes calm blue, or gray, or green, to me
Your eyes are like the ocean—dangerously.

The sonnet pleased me—precisely Shakespearean, with its three quatrains and resolution in a final couplet—but I didn't show it to Martha. It implied more commitment than I meant to make. We were going our different ways for the summer. I knew she had a birthday coming up and decided to send her a small, leather-bound selection of Wordsworth's poems that I'd bought at the university store, writing on the fly-leaf not my sonnet, but some other lines that seemed to me cautiously ambiguous.

Receiving my gift, Martha wrote back with happy appreciation. I was in the New Hampshire woods camping with Elwyn Smith—we were at work on a project of building a log cabin—when Martha's letter reached me. After several days I wrote back, we exchanged a few more messages, and the summer slipped away.

5

I Know What You Will Be Coping With

2001

For some months after the shadow first started to pass across our sun, I struggled with Martha's occasional difficulties without knowing the dreaded disease that was causing them. And I thought—or hoped—that the lapses weren't noticeable. Although I had retired, Martha was still playing the organ for the community church; and after a friend had to give up directing the Rossmoor Chorus—of which I was a member—she took charge of that, too.

So it happened one evening, after rehearsal, another singer spoke privately to me. Her husband, as I knew, was a fairly advanced dementia victim. Sometimes he came with her to rehearsal and sat in the shadows at the back of the auditorium.

This particular evening she was by herself, and most of the others had left. Passing me by on her way out, she said to me, keeping her voice low, "Time to get home to look after my three-year-old." She paused and added, "I know what you will be coping with. I'm sorry."

Just like that. Before I could think of anything to reply, she had left. Clearly, someone was noticing and realizing a change in Martha.

∽∾

I needed advice to help me understand what was happening. I turned to our family doctor, a kind Filipino-American who was never in a hurry with his patients. He suggested an appointment with a neurologist and also an MRI brain scan.

Martha didn't object to the scan. Did she know what was implied? I'm sure she didn't, as I really didn't either. I had some notions of dementia, including my mother's experience with Dad and my own visits with him in a continuing care facility in California a couple of years before he died. But Alzheimer's disease, specifically, was to me an unknown; nor did our doctor talk with us about why the MRI test should be run. He just encouraged Martha to do it, and I supported him.

She hated it. This was the earlier technology: her head was put inside the mechanical doughnut, and she felt all shut in; then the whirring and banging began, accompanied by unbearable noise. Whatever the procedure had accomplished when it was finally over, she declared that she would never submit to it again.

The neurologist, when he saw the pictures of Martha's brain, must have read whatever cues there were, but he did not signal any alarm. He was very low-keyed, even casual. After the appointment he wrote a letter to Martha, noting that she was functioning well.

30

He would be glad to see her again when she might wish, but for the present, his treatment would be "benign neglect." Perhaps this was his calculated approach: we didn't know what he may have communicated to our family doctor—only that neither of them made a mention of Alzheimer's.

6

How God Meant It to Be

1940

With that spring date in Princeton, I had really come to see Martha as the charmingly vivacious person she was. Then we'd gone our separate ways for the summer. Back there in early fall, we met and talked two or three times.

Westminster—still short on dormitory space— had arranged with an elderly couple on nearby Moore Street to lodge students in much of their large house, and Martha was one of the lodgers. It was a great arrangement. The couple would withdraw in the evening to their side of the house, leaving the dining and living rooms comfortably available for the college girls to entertain their dates.

The evening of October 8, 1940, was mild, and the air was pleasant. Because two other couples were inside, Martha and I sat on the front porch. I'd seen her two or three times since early September, riding my bicycle across town from the seminary. My fellowship in English that included residence in the university's graduate college was just for a year; now I was starting preparation for the ministry at Princeton Theological Seminary. That evening, the bicycle was leaning against the step rail in the warm dark as we talked, and a late moon began to show through the trees.

Suddenly, Martha was telling me what she had thought through the summer; how she felt about me. It came out in a rush, her frankness and trust leaving me moved and shaken. I found her deeply appealing; but was I ready to reciprocate? What would that mean for both of us and our future?

"Let's give ourselves three days," I proposed. "We won't see each other; we won't talk any more for that time. It will help us know what God has for us."

I felt the weight of the decision I needed to make. Martha seemed decided, but that only added to my responsibility. I was more than three years older and already in seminary. And we would be taking each other's lives in our hands, a commitment that would be for a lifetime. I rode back to the seminary that night, hardly seeing the streets or how I got there.

I needed to pray, to come to see, as I believed, how God meant our relationship to be. Martha and I were both anchored in a devout, evangelical Christian faith. As I sat through lectures the next day, my mind and my intention were to be open to the Spirit. What happened was a quieting, an inward assurance replacing my misgivings. There was no vision, no startling sign from heaven—just that calm assurance that what was happening was right. By late afternoon, I phoned Martha to say I'd like to come that evening—after all, did we need the full three days?

In my sparse dormitory room at the seminary in the evening dusk, I made a sort of preparation. I read again from Genesis the story of Jacob's love for Rachel and his commitment to her. Then I put on my phonograph a record of Tchaikovsky's Fifth Symphony, filling my room with the rousing, confident Fourth Movement. These were a sufficient send-off; they lifted me and my bicycle through shadows toward Moore Street and Martha.

She met me, and not many words were needed. Again we were together on the porch in warm, early October darkness. I held her close and said, "I know now that I love you. I always will." We committed ourselves to each other—for life. She was only eighteen, a beginning sophomore in college, but she had decided. She declared to me that she had no doubts.

Next day, in the university store, I chose a small gold ring with the Princeton shield and had it engraved inside: *MCB.DRF.10.9.40.* I put it on her finger. On a weekend at home some days later, as she told me, she rolled the ring across the kitchen table, giving her parents the news.

Henry Bradway commented, "Well, he seems to be a good man, sincere, and he'll be a Presbyterian minister—not so sure about that Presbyterian part (said with a twinkle, as he liked to do); but we'll leave that for down the road, if and when it comes time to think about a wedding."

Della's comment was more direct, and cautious: "He's older than you are, and quite a bit further along. I hope you can keep up with him."

Martha answered that she wouldn't try to keep up. She'd make her own way—which, over the years, she did.

Three days after Martha and I made our commitment to each other, I put my ponderings into a sonnet. We had come from far-separated beginnings. That had to be expressed in an ocean image—"the wind that brought such wanderers here across the dawning sea." I couched my concluding conviction in terms of evangelical faith—that was my way of putting it at that time. I'd say it somewhat differently now, but the conviction of rightness in our relationship would be the same seventy years later.

Martha

When in the secret shadow of my thought
I wonder at the love you have for me,
And try to understand the wind that brought
Such wanderers here across the dawning sea,
We two, who scarcely could have thought to be
Together and alone, who never sought
This quiet beach under the quiet lee,
But yet are here; then comes deep-sinking
    thought
To say, raising my eyes beyond the line
Where water burns into the morning sky,
"Believe you God—the hands that intertwine,
Pierced in his love, the silver cord? On high
He loves you both; why ask a further sign
That he has willed your love? It shall not die."

7

Banana Cream Pie

2001

It had been clear to most of our children and grandchildren that Martha was not managing things as capably as she was used to doing. Although this was more noticeable at gatherings at what we called the Bay House, even there the family simply attributed to advancing age any slips that Mom or Grandma made.

The Bay House—what happy memories! Martha and I bought it almost on a whim. I was looking for a place to keep and to sail *Por Fin*, the sailboat I had finally (*por fin* in Spanish) finished building in our garage. We went prospecting around the eastern shore of the upper Chesapeake Bay, ran across this modest bungalow offered at a good price, went back in late afternoon to see it again, and called and made our bid when we returned home that evening. Over the years, we added to the house until it could sleep eighteen or twenty people. It became a summer haven for Donna's family, crossing the country from California. Her husband, Eric, enjoyed the peace and freedom of cycling many miles on country roads, and the children, Erica, Jessica and Fletcher, spent hours on the beach and in the water. The Bay House also became a joyous rounding-up place for larger family groups, particularly during Christmas.

A festive memory: our holiday cluster standing around the piano, trying out the harmonies as Martha took us through a few Christmas hymns, then led us caroling around the neighborhood, all bundled up brightly, she giving us our pitches in the frosty air.

At the Bay House, Martha was—and liked to be—in charge. It was the way she had been brought up, the way her mother had behaved in their house. Martha planned the meals, saw to it that supplies were on hand, and set the meal hours. That third chore was a trial. Breakfast could hardly be controlled. There were those in the family who liked to talk late into the night, perhaps over a glass of wine, so that next morning Martha, having made breakfast and cleaned up the kitchen, would keep finding more cereal bowls and coffee cups left around later and later in the day.

Dinner, at the least, must be punctual with everyone gathering and sitting down together. If 6:30 p.m. was agreed on, then 6:30 p.m. it should be. Martha, busy at the kitchen range readying a large, bubbling pot for corn-on-the-cob or whatever else she was cooking, might recruit as messenger a grandchild who happened by:

"Alex, go down to the beach and tell Granddad and the others that it's six o'clock. They'd all better be coming up to get ready for dinner."

So Alex would appear at the strip of the beach, where it shelves into the cool, brackish water of the Sassafras River mouth on the upper Chesapeake Bay. This was only a hundred yards from our house, cutting through the downhill neighbors' yard by agreement. The beach is coarse, gray sand and nasty burrs lurk in the grass, a hazard for bare feet; but it looks across sparkling water to Ordinary Point, a quarter-mile away. Much nearer, in wading distance at low tide, my sailboat would be riding at its anchor buoy.

"Grandma says it's almost dinnertime and you'd all better come up and get ready."

Alex is Marilyn and Dale's daughter. When our son-in-law Dale visited the Bay House, he would come provided with a cooler stocked with beer and sodas for the beach. In younger years I was a strict teetotaler; but by this stage I'd enjoy a glass of wine or an occasional gin and tonic mix, and definitely a cold beer on the beach.

Dale might respond to Alex's message with, "We'll be along. You can tell Grandma we were getting things together, but that it's Granddad who's holding us up. He just took another beer, and we have to wait for him to finish it."

That wouldn't be true; but Dale knew how Martha felt, brought up by a mother who wore the white ribbon of the Women's Christian Temperance Union. Although Martha had come to accept the family's beer, wine, and cocktails in moderation, they still made her a bit uncomfortable and created an invitation for Dale's playful humor.

Let me go on reconstructing a Bay House scene as it might have been at this time in Martha's transition. In the kitchen up the hill, she has just started to ease shucked ears of corn into her boiling pot when Janice comes up from a basement bedroom. Looking into the kitchen, she quickly notes a problem.

"Mom,"—although a daughter-in-law, it's in Janice's nature to use Mom and Dad rather than our first names—"what beautiful corn! Did that come from the farm stand at the main road?"

"I think so."

"It must have been picked just yesterday or even this morning. Here, let's wait a few minutes before it goes into the water. I heard you speaking to Alex. The beach crowd will be coming up, but it always takes them awhile."

While talking, Janice has found a pair of tongs and has been retrieving the two or three ears already bobbing in the pot. "This way your beautiful corn will be fresh and straight out of the boiling water when we're all sitting around the table," she adds.

Martha has drawn back a little, but makes no objection. Janice goes on, "I'd had enough sun and came up to get showered. I could help with the salad. I see that Dad and Tom got tomatoes, cucumbers, and lettuce along with the corn."

Down at the beach, the group has begun to fold beach chairs and pile towels on the cooler. I climb the slope ahead of them to give Martha reassurance. I am feeling vaguely guilty that I've been down at the water, relaxing, and want to be ready to help, maybe making sure that enough places are set and with sufficient flatware. When I get there, I find that Marilyn, who left before I did, has already unobtrusively exchanged and rearranged a few things, signaling to me that all is well.

On this day, there were two places to be added. In the afternoon on the beach, we'd had the fun of watching for Larry's sailboat to appear beyond Ordinary Point. Son Larry is the one of our six who inherited my love of sailing. He also inherited his father-in-law's boat—a 22-foot cruising sailboat similar to mine. This time, he and his older son, Paul, were crossing the Bay from Baltimore. With a fickle wind, the crossing could be an all-day sail, and as it happened, Larry and Paul had to do much of it under power. They came around the point with sails set, but needed the outboard to make a landing on the beach.

After dinner, the long, cool evening is to be enjoyed.

"Let's take a boat ride," I propose. "It looks like we'll have a beautiful sunset."

"Sure," Martha responds. "You go along, all who want to. I'll stay and tidy up a few things here."

Tom protests, "No, Mom, not a bit. You've done more than enough already; now you need to enjoy the sunset out on the water."

"I don't think so. I can see it from here."

"Come, Mom," Janice joins in. "we need you, to make it a party."

Together, we convince her. I bring the sailboat alongside the landing at the little pier that runs out into the water from the beach. Tom and Janice help Martha aboard. With the outboard motor purring at low speed, we move out on painted water in an evening calm. Our voices and laughter drift across it, to where tree branches trail on the further shore. Guiding the motor, I reach my free hand to squeeze Martha's. The stress lines in her face have softened. In the west, some streaks of cloud burn gold at the lower edges, and ruddy light bathes our faces. I glance at the other passengers, around and beyond Martha. They are part of the family we have been given, and I have her here, my love, out on the water. Its richly stained ripples wash and baptize my spirit.

"Let's sing 'Day Is Dying in the West' just the first stanza," I propose. The hymn has special associations for me from my childhood in Korea, and the family knows it as a favorite.

Tom says, "Mom, give us the pitch."

Abruptly, Martha starts to sing. The pitch is obviously too high; but we all join in, straining at the high notes near the end. Even Larry, used to singing tenor, has to shift to falsetto. It hurts to remember how musically accurate Martha always was.

Later, with all the ending procedures done—passengers disembarked, the boat moored again, the gear secured for the night—we are on the porch of our house. In gathering dusk, the young people are merrily running and calling, playing a game of kick the can. Among them are Tom and Janice's college daughter, Megan—half gazelle, who likes to run on country roads—and Christine, a late high-schooler already fascinated by marine biology. Marilyn and Dale's Andy, three years older than Alex, joins in, too.

These kids are too old for a children's game, all except Paul and maybe Alex, but it is a nostalgic part of vacationing at the Bay House. On the porch, I feel that Martha is happy, and I am happy, hearing the voices and watching the swift shadows of swallows crisscrossing the lawn and the glimmering sparks of fireflies among the trees.

∞∞

At that time, the family was still attributing Martha's occasional difficulties simply to her age. Even I was, I suppose, somewhat in denial, not recognizing that the encroaching shadow was, in fact, Alzheimer's.

There was the incident of Tom's birthday pie, also at the Bay House. The pie went back to Tom's early years. He was Tommy then, about seven or eight years old, and we were living in Mexico City. Tommy loved that dessert. On very special occasions we would go to Shirley Courts, an American-style restaurant, and Tommy could order their banana cream pie. It was so special for him that when we were leaving Mexico, Martha persuaded the chef to give her the recipe. Each year for Tom's birthday she would make the dessert, learning to turn it out to perfection—the custard layer and fruit-and-cream layers piled high with a deep, fluffy meringue, delicately browned under a broiler.

For August 21, 2001, Tom's 50th birthday, the family staged a major celebration at the Bay House. It even included a trek to Baltimore arranged by Larry, so that we could see the Orioles, Tom's favorite baseball team, in a game. But back at the Bay House the climax of dinner, the banana cream pie, did not turn out. The layers didn't rise as they should. The meringue lay limply on top, refusing to fluff up and to brown. Something had happened to Martha's master touch, although no one was willing to say so. The rest of the family could only pretend not to notice what a sad, soggy representation this was of Shirley Courts' wonderful pie.

8

In the Valparaiso
Railroad Café

1942, 1945, 1946

Martha was still in her teens when we were married on May 19, 1942—three weeks later she turned twenty. For the wedding in the classically colonial First Presbyterian Church in Princeton, her attendants carried candles. Some had protested, but Martha was adamant. What we were saying and doing was before God, asking God's blessing on it. The candles would be part of that.

And they were. Outside, it was a bright spring evening; but in the shadowy sanctuary each attendant's face took the warm, flickering light, and together, they formed a reverent tableau.

Then Martha herself was moving down the aisle—radiant, sweetly solemn in the focus of her mind. Wearing sculpted, white satin, she held in a hand that trembled just a little a Bible in white covers that trailed lilies of the valley on its ribbons. Her other hand was on her father's arm. Henry Bradway was bringing his daughter down the aisle—the ultimate tribute of his fatherhood. When they reached the front, he stepped around and I joined Martha, facing him. In his more familiar clergy role, Henry began to speak the service, although at first it took some effort to control his voice.

We had memorized our vows; that was important. The words were traditional, but we weren't just repeating them. Looking into each other's eyes, we made our commitment for always.

After the words, scriptures, and prayers, the Westminster Choir themselves—a special honor— sang the school's signature "Lutkin Benediction". Its soaring cadence built and built, filling every crevice of the sanctuary, then subsided, leaving a last, serenely poignant amen to float away in late spring twilight.

∽∾

After our wedding, Martha finished her major in organ at Westminster Choir College and went on to a master's in musicology. Completing a graduate year in English at the university, I had turned to training for the ministry at Princeton Theological Seminary. Exempt from the draft, I had considered applying to become a navy chaplain (the army required pastoral experience), but decided, rather, on missionary service. Martha and I submitted our application to the Presbyterian Board of Foreign Missions. They assigned us to Chile—said they had the very place for us, working with students at the University of Chile in Santiago.

This was an adventure—more so for Martha, who had not been out of the United States. We left Miami before dawn, soaring out over the Caribbean in the sunrise in a huge propeller plane. Before noon, we were changing flights in Barranquilla, Colombia, then were dropped down in the lush, green valley of Medellin by mid-afternoon. Our home for six months of intensive Spanish study would be a middle-class house built around a central patio—no doors and no glass windows, just shutters opening in and iron grillwork outside for security. Medellin's perpetual springtime invited openness—with tiled floors throughout the house and large, tropical cockroaches based in the kitchen area that came foraging at night.

We were beginning to get a grip on the language and to feel at home in the culture when we moved far south to Santiago, Chile. The year that followed was disconcerting, although it started idyllically. We arrived to a huge celebration of Protestant Christians (the preferred term in Spanish is *evangélicos*) in a central park. It had been exactly a century since the arrival in Valparaiso of David Trumbull—a Presbyterian minister and the first Protestant missionary to Chile.

But as we got our feet on the ground, we began to be aware of a deep rift between the Presbyterian mission, of which we were a part, and the leadership of the small, struggling churches that formed the Presbytery of Chile. The mission controlled the use of funding that came from the Board in New York, and therefore controlled some important schools and institutions, while the presbytery, with only its small churches, felt side-lined. That year, as new arrivals, we found ourselves being made a test case. The presbytery leadership declared that they had no interest in a university-student work in Santiago. In the end, they put forward an ultimatum:

"We want the Fletchers to serve the church in Vallenar, or we want them nowhere in Chile."

We flew to Vallenar, some four hundred miles north of Santiago—a drab, brown city with bits of dusty green spread on the floor of a narrow valley in the country's rainless northern region. The people who were apparently the principal family, among a half dozen forming the congregation, received us warmly. They had prepared a room for us, likely the best that they had.

That night, Martha lay awake. Right over her head, seeming like a few inches away, would come a screech and scuffle between the bare ceiling and the corrugated tin roof above it. She got out of bed to put on the light—she had to have light. The single bulb hanging from the ceiling showed a bare floor—no sign of rats—and the scuffling overhead had stopped. But the situation still felt hopeless. Everything was so drab and depressing: the plain, adobe house fronts along the dusty street and the little church building with its dusty bell.

Daunting as an assignment in Vallenar seemed, I probably would have attempted it, but Martha declared it impossible. After the year's tensions in Santiago, she appeared already near the edge of a nervous collapse. We went back to Santiago, to the mission's executive committee, with our dilemma. The committee of our colleagues had no solution, no help to offer. We would have to work out with presbytery whatever we could.

Some days later, we were sitting at a small table in the café of the Valparaiso railroad station. Across from us was the Chilean pastor who was that year's moderator of the Presbytery of Chile. Face to face, we found him kind and sympathetic. But he pointed out to us that we must understand his position. We did, and in that damp and drafty station, we worked out a compromise: Martha and I would leave Santiago and go north to serve the church, as the presbytery wished, but we'd go much further north than Vallenar. It would be to Antofagasta, chief city of northern Chile and eight hundred miles away. There, we would undertake to found an entirely new Presbyterian church program.

9

Just Stay With
Your Cue Cards

2001

I wrote a play to be put on under the auspices of Rossmoor Community Church. I was retired from the pastorate and my long hospital stay was behind me. The play, called *Passion: 2001*, would propose a setting of the gospel's passion story in contemporary Jerusalem. The Jesus figure (not to appear on stage) would be Yeshua, an Israeli from Galilee. I had a good time with other characters, bringing in Mary, Martha, and Lazarus—siblings in the gospel story, whom I cast as Palestinian Americans who had returned to the land of their parents to make a life for themselves in Jerusalem. And for the real life Martha I had a special role, that of Maddy (Miriam Madeleine), an American tourist/archeologist, standing for the biblical Mary Magdalene.

In the play Maddy meets up by chance with Lazarus (Laz), who brings her home to meet his sisters. There she hears about the charismatic Yeshua. Her response is immediate: "I want to meet him. Do you think there's a chance I could meet him?"

She does, and she becomes involved in his story. He has come from Galilee to Jerusalem, leading an impromptu demonstration to urge compassionate understanding among Jews, Muslims, and Christians. So it comes about that the next morning Maddy is outside a synagogue with Laz and a small crowd, waiting for Yeshua to emerge, when she witnesses his assassination. All of this takes place off stage, but Madeleine has a vivid, crucial speech when she bursts into the apartment to tell the horrified sisters, Mary and Martha, what has happened. Here is the last part of her story.

> Laz jumped forward, but I grabbed his arm. The assassins—they had vanished. There was Sy (Simon Peter), down on his knees beside Yeshua, holding him, sobbing—and then the white coats putting him in an ambulance— flashing lights, wailing sirens—gone—and just that red, red blood on the sidewalk. Oh, God, God!

I wrote the part for Martha, being sure she could make it real. In act three, scene one, it is morning in the apartment a couple of days later. Maddy, up early, has gone alone to Yeshua's tomb for a final visit before she leaves to return to America. The others are gathered, subdued and depressed.

Maddy enters, her face mystical, radiant. In several bursts, against the surprise and disbelief of the others, she recounts her experience—finding the marble slab pulled away and the tomb empty, sobbing alone in the garden, becoming aware of someone standing near, hearing her name spoken, and knowing that it is Yeshua.

The part was a good fit for Martha—a sort of Anne of Green Gables grown up, innocent, almost naïve, but capable of swift and passionate dedication. The trouble was that in rehearsal some of her key lines kept coming out garbled, disconnected. This was Rossmoor, a senior community. Memorizing could be difficult, so the cast had cue cards they could use both in rehearsal and performance.

"Martha," I was saying, "you have some long speeches. Don't worry about them. Just stay with your cue cards; read them, if you need to. You can do it with feeling and expression, but it's important to have the lines clear, exactly as they're written."

Did she understand me? She would nod in agreement, but even in the final performance some of the lines were moved around and some came out ad-libbed in a confusing way. I was deeply disappointed, and also troubled. I'd thought that Martha could play the part with wonderful effect the way she used to be able to do. She didn't make any apology after the play was over. She was apparently unaware of having gotten anything wrong. I could only hold back from saying more about it; just remember not to try any more dramatic roles.

☙❧

Not long afterward, Martha said she was going to resign as organist of the church. She was tired of the pressure. The job included arranging the weekly booking for a professional soloist, who then had to be accompanied. Was she realizing that these coordinating tasks were becoming more difficult? Was playing unfamiliar music accompaniments that had to be sight-read, which used to be routine for her, now becoming a challenge?

Perhaps she had decided to step aside before she was asked to. I didn't ask if that was her thinking, but I agreed with the decision, feeling relief that we would avoid the risk of some awkward and embarrassing crisis. We weren't talking about her problem, even without the Alzheimer's name attached to it. I could only conjecture as to how aware of it she might be.

10

The Other Discovery

1947

We did it—Santiago to Antofagasta, in the well-worn car the mission designated for our use. That was a thousand miles of dirt-and-gravel road—the Pan-American Highway, winding over low mountains, then straightening out across the endless, rocky desert of northern Chile. In the car were three of us, Orfelina, Martha, and I. Orfelina had been our rather emotional home aide for our year in Santiago. She wanted to go with us on the trip north.

We had no idea—as we rattled and jarred over the washboard surface that dirt roads develop in the desert—that Orfelina was pregnant. That was one discovery that she admitted to us in the kitchen of the rambling guest bungalow in Antofagasta that was our temporary lodging. The other discovery, one that took a little longer to become evident, was that Martha, too, had been pregnant for all those thousand rugged miles. We'd been married for almost five years. Now for Martha, along with everything else new in our venture in this desert seaport, there was going to be a first pregnancy and anticipated motherhood. As for Orfelina, we convinced her that she needed to go back to her husband, riding the narrow-gauge railroad for forty-eight hours back to Santiago.

For the new project in our new location, we had—as an entering wedge—a letter to a local judge. He was a graduate of the prestigious Presbyterian Boys' Academy in Santiago and was known to be sympathetic to our cause. The judge put us in touch with the owner of Antofagasta's radio station, who gave us a free quarter-hour slot during Sundays at noon.

A few readers may remember the Estey folding organ. Each Sunday, we would drive far up one of the bare slopes overlooking the city and its port. There we would lug our Estey by its carrying handle into the tin-roofed building—not much more than a shack—that stood by the transmission tower and served as a provisional studio. Seated at the organ, Martha would work its pedals to keep the organ's bellows full, as she played and sang close into a microphone. It was remarkable how mellow the metal reeds of the organ sounded over the air. I would have a Bible reading and a brief message. To get our name known, we called our program *La Hora Presbiteriana*, the Presbyterian Hour. A special reward for us, as we made our spoken Spanish as natural as we could, was to have an occasional radio listener express surprise on learning that it was North American gringos whom he or she had been hearing on the *Hora Presbiteriana*. Later, we changed the name to *Oasis del Alma*, The Soul's Oasis. That was when we had brought back from the United States a Hammond electronic organ and one of the early tape recorders and had graduated to a half-hour program that we could tape in advance.

Martha flew to Santiago to have her baby. Some friends joked about the apparent effect on her of the northern *salitre*, the nitrate mined in the desert that is a potent natural fertilizer, but we knew that baby Donna had started on the way just before we set out for what Chileans call the Norte Grande, the Great North of the formidable Atacama Desert.

I've been looking again at a cherished photo I have of Martha and little Donna, not yet two, in the central island of the avenue close to where we were living. It was a favorite spot because, unlike most of Antofagasta's dry streets, this one contained greenery that the municipality kept watered. Martha is standing beside the bulging, clipped trunk of a pineapple palm, with Donna on a high step. A snug blue sweater and a plaid, wool skirt set off Martha's dark hair and show her as slim at 27 as she was when I first met her. The bright plaid of her skirt is repeated in Donna's jumper, and Donna wears a matching blue sweater. Martha had made both plaid outfits on her tabletop sewing machine.

11

Lasagna in an Oven Drawer?

2004, 2005

"Martha, what happened to that leftover lasagna?"
"I put it away."
"Put it away where?"
"There in the kitchen."

The lasagna wasn't in the refrigerator where it ought to be, nor in the pantry, nor the oven.

"Look in the oven; maybe I left it in there."
"I did; no lasagna in the oven."

Then a thought—the drawer at the bottom of the range. Sure enough, there was the casserole with leftover lasagna, stored away on top of another casserole dish and several pans. Far more disconcerting was that a back burner on the stove was on and red hot. Had it been left on all morning?

I cringed, troubled that I hadn't seen it sooner, imagining thin tongues of flame reaching the cabinets beside and above the range. I'd need to watch over some of the cooking and housekeeping as casually as possible. This should include loading the washing machine. In our bungalow, the washer and dryer were in a closet off the hallway. We had already experienced one almost-flood, when too large a load with too much detergent sent soapy water sloshing onto the carpet.

Driving was also a potential worry. Fortunately, Martha was used to having me drive whenever we went anywhere together. Now, I would just offer to go along when there was grocery shopping or some other errand to be done. She seemed satisfied to have it that way. She still carried her set of car keys in her handbag—no need to make an issue by asking her to give them up. I just took care that she didn't use them.

I did arrange a consultation with our family doctor—just a routine thing, I told Martha. He ran through a sort of basic mental status examination, and asked some twenty questions: What day of the week was it? What county were we living in? Who was currently the President of the United States? She got the day right, but missed the county—not surprisingly, I thought. Who pays much attention to counties? She also missed on the president—more of a lapse.

After some other questions, the doctor said, "I'd like you to copy the drawing I'm making."

He proceeded to draw a pentagon in simple straight lines, then a second one overlapping the first. Martha took the pencil and drew in the blank space that the doctor indicated—two figures, also with five sides and overlapping, roughly similar to his shapes. The doctor's figure had looked complicated to me, so I felt surprise and relief when Martha was able to copy it with all the essential features.

He commended her, giving me an unspoken sign that she had done well. He did give her a prescription for Aricept—"Something you might find helpful; but be sure to let me know if it seems to have any unpleasant side effects," he said. At that time Aricept didn't yet have a particular significance for me, as a medication for Alzheimer's patients, and it had no apparent side effects on Martha. She generally tolerated any medication.

∞∞

We had a vacation house in Brick Township on the Jersey shore—a reinvestment of funds from the sale of the Bay House. It was a charming little bungalow located at a juncture of lagoons that gave us a pleasing view northwest down one waterway. The lagoons are a network of canals dug so that the tidal water of Barnegat Bay fills them, and boats moored at their docks can motor out to the open bay.

There was one family roundup here—at what we began to call the Shore House—soon after we bought it. After that, it was mostly I who urged using it. Martha would go along when I wanted to drive down for some days in the summer or a night or two in winter—the house had very efficient gas heat—but she never shared my enthusiasm.

I remember one December evening, soon after dark, when we were leaving the house to drive back to Rossmoor. Christmas was coming on, and up and down our short street neighbors, including those next door on our right, had strung up holiday lights. Coming out the front door, Martha stopped on the porch to look around.

"Let's go over there," she said, indicating the house facing us. I objected that we didn't really know those people and shouldn't be trespassing. She went down the few steps with me toward our car, but then started to pull my arm. She wanted to go up the street where there were more lights, maybe to see somebody. As I urged that we get in the car, she fixed her attention on that house next door, to the right. I had talked with the pleasant young couple who lived there, meeting them casually as they worked around their yard. Now Martha was determined; she had to ring their bell and go inside. What should I do? I could hardly seize her and force her into our car. Better to count on our friends' understanding, and let her have her way.

When Kathy, our neighbor, opened the door, there was a rush of warmth, lights, and the sound of voices. She already had visitors, but Martha pushed in eagerly. Her response to Kathy's surprised welcome was off the mark, as each statement or question continued to be. I tried to cover, and I was glad that Kathy quickly took in the situation. She led us into the living room, introducing her guests, while Martha was quite conversational without really connecting most of the time.

All this was more than I had bargained for on agreeing to let Martha ring the doorbell. It was a relief, but at the same time, it was painful to realize that several others in the room, as well as Kathy, were quick to grasp how it was with Martha. They responded to her as if she were making complete sense while Kathy seated her in a comfortable chair, offering tea or coffee and a piece of the pie they had recently been sharing. I hastily assured Kathy that we had looked in for just a minute and needed to be on our way—feeling, acutely, how odd our visit had to appear.

I let a few minutes pass, trying to act natural in such an unnatural situation. Then I took Martha's hand to get her out of the chair and move toward the door with effusive thanks to Kathy, and best holiday wishes to all. How glad I felt when we were once more out in the chill of the night, and when I had Martha unprotestingly buckled into her car seat beside me! But Kathy's kindness and that of her friends, accepting my wife as a person with a crippling disability, brought a sharp pang I knew I would have to get used to in more social encounters in the future.

⚭⚭

Our kitchen in Rossmoor looked across a patch of inside lawn with some flowers on each side in summer, directly into the kitchen of our neighbors and close friends. And, because JoAnne, the neighbor, lit a candle in her window when she was making dinner, Martha began doing the same. It became a wordless reaching across the small space, a tradition we kept up for many months. Then, I began to notice that Martha would leave her candle unlit. When I remarked about it, finding a fresh candle and lighting it for her, she showed little interest. In time, there was no small flickering light from our side.

12

Pastor, Pastor, Help Me!

1949–1956

O ur Antofagasta venture had its ups and downs. I
can picture Martha in our improvised chapel in
a property we rented on a significant street. Opening
onto the sidewalk, it had a deep room designed for a
shop or small business, with an apartment above. We
adapted the deep room to be a youth center, with short
chapel pews at one side; there we held a weekly worship
service for anyone who would come.

In my mental picture, Martha is sitting at the Estey
organ, pumping the pedals to play a hymn, while little
Donna has climbed into her lap. In the pews are one or
two high school students, drawn to our youth center,
and an older woman in a black shawl. They make up my
congregation as I stand at the lectern to lead worship.

❧

Fast forward about five years. After Donna came Sylvia.
For this birth Martha opted to stay in Antofagasta,
using the low, strung-together Spanish colonial
hospital. Attended by a skilled midwife, she went
through labor and delivery in a private room whose
only door opened directly on a flagstone patio. There,

Donna and I waited out a long afternoon; she running around, exploring some large potted plants and wanting to know why Mommy was behind that closed door. Finally, with tremulous excitement, we heard that first cry through the muffling door, and after what seemed a long while, the door opened. We went in carefully to see Mommy holding a bundle with a small, red-faced baby—Donna's sister, Sylvia.

In those five years, we also had a leave in the United States for study and for promoting support for our work. Near the end of that leave, Tommy made his entrance, helped by a stateside obstetrician and modern hospital facility. Back in Antofagasta, we moved to a beautiful property that had been a well-known restaurant and a commercial vegetable garden. There, we planned and built a pastor's house and a home for high school girls coming from mining camps up on the *pampa*—where only elementary schooling was available.

∞∞

Occupying the pastor's house, we found our personal and professional lives in constant interaction every day. I set up an office in a surviving part of the former restaurant. Martha supervised her household and three young children, while sharing in the activities of our nascent church. About a year after we returned from stateside leave, she was pregnant again; we would be adding a fourth child, presumably another Antofagasta birth.

Then Martha miscarried. Her pregnancy was not far advanced, just at the end of the second month or early in the third. At the hospital, when the doctor had finished attending her, he came out to me.

"Are you a strong man?" he asked. "Do you want to see?"

When I said yes, he carefully brought out in his gloved hand a small mass of flesh, seemingly shapeless, saying, "You see, that is all."

Martha and I were both shaken by the miscarriage. I took her home—we were just two blocks from the hospital—to rest in our first-floor guest room, avoiding the stairs. In my office, under the emotion of the day, I began to write. A lyric took form, and I carried it back to the house. Finding Martha alone in that downstairs bedroom, I read the poem to her with as much control as I could manage. We held each other for a long time, after the shaking emotion subsided.

Here is the lyric, "To Our Child Unborn", written in Antofagasta, a desert city with unwashed streets overlooked by bare, unchanging hills—a place where it almost never rains.

> Across the placid infinite you came
> Like a line of light thrown from a floating star,
> Too far, too thin and tenuous to see
> Shine out and fade; you never had a name,
> Child that was to be.
> And now you're gone, they say we should not
> grieve;
> That it's no loss, because you were not born;
> Because your soul flashed by, a meteorite
> That grazed this atmosphere and dropped again
> Into the sun-strewn infinite. What then?

Shall we shrug off so great a thing—just nod,
And take the chilly, clinical word of fact,
A bit of flesh inanimate? My soul
Is not more soul than yours. I breathe this air
You never breathed, earth-bound; but now it
    chokes,
It sickens me; my eyes fill up. O star,
O faint, brief star, soul of my soul, how far
Will you out-distance and out-beckon me,
Child that was to be?
My heart is calmer now; we shall go on;
Here in this world of time all must go on.
But she and I will not forget, and we
Will lift for you an unseen monument
Beyond the noisome streets, the rainless hills,
Beyond the thought of all this little earth,
Against the courses of the reeling stars
We'll write your name, who never had a name.
Grief of two hearts will be your elegy,
Child that was to be.

The culminating phase of construction, coming near the end of our time in Antofagasta, was the planning and erection of a gracious church building having some touch of Spanish-style architecture, set prominently on our street corner. This brought us to a climactic evening—the dedication service for the permanent home of Christ the King Presbyterian Church. For this service I wanted something unusual and memorable; something that would say dramatically what the church was meant to be in that community. Taking a leaf from the morality plays of late medieval England and counting on the Latin flair for the dramatic and symbolic that was part of the Chilean culture, I wrote and prepared a sermon to be acted out, including symbolic figures.

As the service began, some members of our congregation knew what friends and well-wishers from other Protestant churches in the city did not know—that this would not be a usual sort of service, although it started out in the customary way. There were opening hymns and scripture readings; then I took my stand in the new pulpit and began to make welcoming remarks.

Abruptly, a man looking like a disheveled laborer calls from the back of the sanctuary. "Pastor, Pastor, help me!"

Some of the people, assuming he is drunk, tell him to be quiet and try to hold him back as he starts to push down the crowded aisle. But I call to him,

"What is it, friend? What do you need? Perhaps we can help you here."

Puzzled, people let the laborer pass and he comes forward, pouring out a familiar story of addiction to cheap wine that has cost him jobs and left his wife and children penniless. At the organ, now our richly versatile Hammond, Martha has begun softly a familiar theme hymn, "Just As I Am, Without One Plea", and from beside the chancel, one of our high school girls enters, dressed in white. As I invite the laborer to come up into the chancel, she speaks to him:

"I am Purity. I am what you need. Here in the church, this is what you can find. Give yourself to Christ, and we will help you."

Martha lets the music swell. The laborer kneels, then takes his place beside Purity. I resume the service, but am interrupted by an audible sobbing. A woman, her head covered, moves out of one of the pews, makes her way impulsively up into the chancel, and begins telling her story. It is another familiar one: a man—he seemed like a good man—promised her; she gave him herself and all she had, then he was gone. Her family won't have her back. She has thought of drowning herself in the cold, black water.

The figure in white who enters across from her—another of our girls—explains that she is Trust. Here the woman can find trust again, trust in God who never fails, and trust among believers, who will support and cherish her.

So it continues—three more stories, three more symbolic figures, young people in white robes. There is an embittered intellectual skeptic who needs to find Faith, a young man stricken with tuberculosis who is met by Hope, and most appealingly, two children off the street. When they have come up into the chancel, the older child, holding her brother by the hand, speaks to me in a clear treble:

"Please, sir! I don't know about this place, but they said we might find help, my brother and me. We have no parents, and the building where we had a little shelter burned down. Please, is there anything for orphans like we are?"

The white-robed figure who enters for this final encounter is a young man, a leader in our youth group. In a strong baritone, he tells the children that he is Love. God's love is freely given, expressed to us in the warmly personal compassion of Jesus Christ, the Savior. There can be love for them here in the family of the church.

Some words of mine sum up the acted Sermon of Dedication. This is what the church can be—is dedicated to being, however imperfectly—a living, daily expression of the grace of God.

Throughout the simple drama, Martha, with her sensitivity and skill at improvisation, has woven each change of mood into a fabric of music. The service closes with full organ, as the congregation joins in an exultant hymn.

∽∾

A year or so later, the time came for us to leave Antofagasta. The church was strong enough to call and support a Chilean pastor, and I had a new assignment as liaison for Presbyterian work in what was labeled the Caribbean Area. Our family now numbered six with the arrival of baby Marilyn, who had been on the way when we dedicated the church building. We found ourselves lining the rail of a ship in Antofagasta harbor—a most unusual perspective for Martha and me. The ship's horn had let out a stunning blast. Down below, ropes were being let loose. A crack of water appeared between the ship's side and the pier. Donna and Sylvia were peering over the rail beside Martha, with Sylvia on tiptoes to see. I had Tommy, who was leaning out as far as he could, and Maria, our household helper, held little Marilyn securely.

Maria, who'd been with us since our return from the last leave, had asked if she could please go with us to the United States, where the family would be for a year while I started my Caribbean assignment. Did she realize that she would be leaving her family and her country for who could say how long? Yes, she did. Hesitantly, we had agreed and had arranged her passage.

We looked down now at the knot of friends—church people—on the pier, waving as the engines started up with a shudder and the ship began to move. We glanced up at those brown hills that had been the backdrop of our life through seven eventful years, thinking that probably we'd never see them again. I expected that for Martha that part wasn't sad; her sadness stemmed from leaving the group below and the home and its surroundings, where so much effort and emotion had been invested.

Another blast on the horn. We were gliding past the light at the end of the breakwater, and a damp breeze was coming up. Martha wanted to get the younger ones, at least, down to the cabin. I stayed at the stern rail a little longer, watching those Antofagasta hills recede into mist.

13

You Just Want to Get Rid of Everything

2007

Reluctantly, I had to face that it was time to think about a move. We had stayed on contentedly in Rossmoor, our over-55 retirement community, for more than seven years after I retired as pastor of the Community Church. But the progress of Martha's illness was undeniable. I had to acknowledge that it would soon be more than I could manage. We needed to be where we would have more help, and we needed to be near at least one of the children.

That latter choice was easy. Marilyn was the only one living in New Jersey, and she and her family were in the Cherry Hill/Voorhees area, where we had lived for twenty-six years. We knew of several Continuing Care Retirement Communities (CCRC) in the area, but none as close to Marilyn's family as we would like to be. Then she told us about Lions Gate, which had just opened only a mile from their door. We visited, liked the staff people whom we met and the fresh new facilities, particularly the great room, dining rooms, library and other common areas. Within a few days we were on a waiting list.

The wait was not long. We had expected months, perhaps even a year; but in two weeks we had word of four available apartments of the size we had specified. We picked number 248 for its pleasant eastern exposure and second-floor view of grass and a patch of woods. Lions Gate's logo, with its iconic lion's head staring through a sort of gateway, carries the motto Independence—Continuing Care—Jewish Tradition. Some of our children questioned whether we would like the kosher cuisine. We brushed that aside; we had adjusted readily to a variety of fare in our lifetime. The important thing was to have at hand in a friendly, comfortable environment the extra care that we might need. At Lions Gate, one could move—always within enclosed, climate-controlled passages—between the independent-living apartments, common rooms, and assisted-living and skilled-nursing facilities.

In addition, I had approvingly taken note of one detail when we were first being shown around. As we passed a modest, neatly appointed room in the common area, our escort had said, "And this is the chapel of all faiths." I liked that, and when we met the friendly, engaging chaplain rabbi, I liked him, thinking to myself that I'd look forward to getting to know him.

⚮

Yet, locating in a CCRC would not be just another move. When we were being shown apartment 248— open and bare as it was—I stood looking out its second floor, living room windows at the ground below, thinking that this would be it. These windows, this view, the whole place would probably define the end phase of life for us. There had always been an expectation that as one phase was finishing, another would begin. Not anymore.

Such realization is slow to sink in. Later, when we'd been at Lions Gate for four years, I joined the Spielers (a.k.a. Drama Club) in putting on a show that borrowed for its opening theme the song "Those Were the Days" from *Cabaret*. At the end of our show, the cast stood together to sing a parody written by one of our members, Bernice.

> These are our days, my friend.
> We know someday they'll end.
> We talk; we sing; we laugh away our fears.
> And, if we're getting fat,
> Well, we can drink to that.
> These are our days, our years, our golden years.

With a few years at Lions Gate, I had come to appreciate the whimsically rueful irony of Bernice's parody.

∽∽∽

Our Rossmoor condo sold rather quickly. Packing for the move was the ordeal. Such downsizing, unavoidable at our time in life, is always difficult. Martha's condition made it that much harder. Alzheimer's diminishes the ability to make choices. That had already begun to be evident eight years earlier, in 1999, when we moved from one house to another in Rossmoor and my delayed recovery from surgery put an extra burden on family members helping to make the transition. But for that move, downsizing was only minimally required.

Now, many choices had to be made; some of them, drastic. We would have dinner provided daily in Lions Gate's pleasant dining rooms. Home cooking would be minimal, and the small kitchen of our apartment offered minimal space for dishes, glassware, and cooking utensils. The difficult choices could be painful for Martha; but it could also be painful for her to feel excluded from the selection process. I tried to include her, without confronting her constantly with decisions of what to do with this or that. Quite often, it meant that I just spirited larger items off to the garage, to a mounting cache that would eventually be loaded and trucked away by the kind people of Trenton Area Rescue Mission.

Packing dishes and glassware, I found, sometimes had to be done twice. When Martha wrapped an item insecurely or put it in the wrong carton, a change needed to be made without seeming to correct her. Keep it cool. We were both stressed; small things could ignite a shower of sparks going something like this:

"What are you doing with those records, and why are you taking them all out?"

"Martha, we've got to empty the entertainment center. The thing is too big; we can't have it in our new apartment."

"I don't care. We've had those records for a long time."

"But we never play them. We use CD's now."

"I don't. You just want to get rid of everything and you don't ask me!" Now the tears were in her voice.

"All right, dear. We'll stack them up here. You can help pick out special ones we can take."

"They're all special. I want all of them!"

I had to let it stop there, and turn her to something else. Later, on my own, I would set aside recordings of Martha's own choirs from University Presbyterian Church in Austin and Trinity Church in Cherry Hill plus a few other special albums. Meanwhile, I found excuses for Martha to spend time with our neighbors and close friends while I pushed toward the moment of intense relief that finally came, when the small moving van was fully loaded and the driver clanged shut its rear door, started his engine, and pulled away.

∽∾∽

At Lions Gate, we found a different life. Our apartment, furnished with familiar objects—bedroom, dining and living room furniture, full-wall bookshelves in the den, and pictures (probably too many) hung on every wall—was meant to feel like home, a reassuring refuge. Martha shared, somewhat, in discussion about what to put where. Decisions regarding cherished items—chiefly pictures and other wall hangings that we'd kept, but now couldn't find space for—were not posed to her. No need to make the move more difficult. Such pieces simply disappeared, to be stowed in Marilyn and Dale's storage locker.

An attractive quality in Martha—partly her nature and partly her upbringing—has always been her outgoing spirit, her ready acceptance of people, whoever they are. Lions Gate has some two hundred residents in the independent-living apartments and cottages. We found ourselves cordially received among them, and with her bright smile and responsiveness when anyone spoke to her, Martha immediately began to endear herself to residents and household staff alike. She didn't remember names, but any friendly gesture was met with a smile and the irresistible lighting up of her wide, blue eyes.

Dinnertime was the prime opportunity for such contacts. Lions Gate keeps arrangements happily informal. The four or five dining rooms flow into one another with a common salad bar and kitchen access. Their tables seat two, four, or six, and can be pushed together for other configurations. We could arrange in advance to sit with other residents, leave that to the hostess, or ask to be seated by ourselves. The servers were young people, many of them students from the high school just up the road. At this stage, Martha would read the menu and make her selection, sometimes with prompting and suggestion. She was also managing her implements at table quite well, although her hands had begun to shake noticeably and small slips from fork or spoon would happen.

Lions Gate had on its staff a gifted and energetic director of activities, who kept things humming. When we got there, there were already groups and clubs of many sorts—catering to whatever interests the residents might have—as well as evening films, lectures, game nights, and more. Martha showed little interest in these things, but then, we had never engaged in the usual bridge-playing groups and had never developed a habit of going to movies, either. She and I did join a spontaneously organized Classical Music Committee that sponsored concerts offered by talented young musicians, and we shared in a successful effort to secure an excellent piano for the stage in the commons hall.

When we left Rossmoor, we had to give up Martha's Wurlitzer organ, which went to Donna in California, and also her rebuilt Steinway grand. By that time, Martha was rarely touching the organ, but I did want to encourage the piano. The hundred-year-old Steinway, valued by a music company just for its shell, sold for enough to replace it with a modest, vertical Essex (a member of the "Steinway family" built in China). I had questioned the idea of buying a piano, feeling it would likely take up space in our small apartment to no purpose, but several of our children were insistent. The instrument, they felt, was so much a part of Martha's identity that a home for her without a piano seemed inconceivable. So, we placed the Essex in our living room at Lions Gate, even though we could only rarely persuade Martha to play it a few minutes at a time. When she did, it was increasingly evident that her fingers could not perform what the brain may have wanted to convey. Watching her could bring a stab of pain, remembering how those supple hands used to dominate the banks of keys and stops of organ consoles they had known.

Our daughter Sylvia made a comment by e-mail that I found very perceptive: "Mom almost never played the piano for her own pleasure. It was always an occupational love or she would play for us children to dance and prance or she would be giving piano lessons to bring in extra money or would use the piano at home to work and think through her organ settings or prepare for a choir rehearsal. Music so defined her as a professional person that, as her faculties diminished, music did not become an alternative hobby."

It's true that Martha did not have any hobby or pastime. Again, Sylvia's perception: "Her work was her life. Caring for the family and learning about new environments, new countries, and new social groups were her hobbies. Even sewing was a utilitarian pastime, which she did with great accomplishment when she had a young family. She always made our matching Easter outfits and in Mexico created elaborate Halloween costumes for all six children with the help of our seamstress."

Martha was neither a reader, nor did she do knitting, crocheting, or any kind of handwork. She wasn't a gardener, nor a collector, although she did like bells and small pitchers. Mostly, she seemed too busy for such hobbies, too focused on her family when the children were younger, and too focused on her work. This was fine, but it left nothing to turn to when work was no longer there and her faculties were beginning to decline.

꩜

At Lions Gate, we came under the care of a young physician who had a specialty in geriatrics. He checked

Martha's physical condition very thoroughly, declaring it good, and approved the medications she was taking. I found him both competent and understanding and felt glad that we were in his hands. The doctor again gave Martha a simplified mental status exam. I noted that she did not do as well as she had earlier with our doctor in Rossmoor. When asked if perhaps we should consult a neurologist, our new doctor gave us a referral to a specialist in nearby Haddonfield. A bit of subterfuge was needed to persuade Martha that we ought to make this visit. I couldn't candidly say we believed we were dealing with Alzheimer's and would like to have the advice of a specialist.

The visit turned out to be disappointing. The specialist, too, asked Martha a series of questions. He had her walk down a corridor unaided, making his observations in a friendly, casual way. Once more, we did not have an explicit diagnosis; but then, would a diagnosis have made any difference? The doctor encouraged Martha to keep on with her medications, and encouraged me to help her stay active and interested. He would be glad to see her again in six months or so. We did go back once, with much the same result. What could or should I have expected? There were medications on the market, such as the Aricept Martha was taking, that might have some effect in slowing the progress of her illness; but there is no wonder drug, no cure. The neurologist could only advise keeping Martha healthy and as active as possible, while exercising due caution against falls.

14

No More Skilled and Dedicated Hands

1956, 1960

My new assignment in the Caribbean Area meant extensive travel, with our family based in the United States for a year and then in Mexico City. In early spring of that first year, there was a landmark conference at Lake Hopatcong in New York State. It drew representatives of Presbyterian churches from around the world. Representing the Caribbean area were delegates from Venezuela, Colombia, Guatemala, and Mexico. Martha and I met them in my new capacity, and we got along so well that we were included in the planning for their part in the final, festive meeting. They wanted to sing *"Las Mañanitas"*, a song popular in all their countries. Martha listened to it a couple of times; then she delighted our new friends as she began to pick out their song on a hotel piano, filling in harmony. Soon they were all joining in exuberantly, and we were fully a part of the group.

☽∞☾

Mexico brought a different experience. We found the culture vibrantly, distinctively different from Chile's. In

Chile, as an illustration, Columbus Day was observed as the *Día de la Raza* or Day of the Race—meaning the white race that had come with such consequence to the Americas. On entering Mexico City, by contrast, we encountered at a major intersection an imposing monument. It was in the form of a Mayan pyramid, with heroic sculptures of figures all bearing distinctly Mayan features. This was the *Monumento a la Raza*, Monument to the Race—the indigenous race. In all of Mexico City, there was not so much as a street named for Hernán Cortés, the Spanish conquistador who altered the country's history.

We came to appreciate the independent vigor of Mexican culture, evident in art and architecture—also evident in the Presbyterian Church of Mexico, stronger and more independent than that of any other Latin American country except Brazil. We began to attend the large Prince of Peace church downtown, joining its Felix Mendelssohn Choir. Then, the dynamic young choir director announced that he was leaving, going to the United States to study choral music—as we were delighted to hear—at Martha's alma mater, Westminster Choir College. He said in his farewell speech that he could think of no more skilled and dedicated hands to which to entrust leadership of his beloved choir than those of Señora Martha Fletcher.

"The honor is mine," she assured him and all the choir members present. "I will do my best to carry forward the tradition of musical excellence in Christian worship you have so effectively begun here." I was proud of her fluency and poise in her acceptance remarks.

❧❧

Our years in Mexico City were memorable. Larry was born there, completing our family. By the time we left Mexico, Donna was entering her teens and she and Sylvia were rather deeply imbued with the Mexican culture. I kept busy in my liaison function, logging many air miles and many days away from home that put most of the domestic burden on Martha. For a while, we had a wonderful rented property—a whimsically designed Spanish colonial house with a second floor that was a sort of turret, having several bedrooms accessed by a winding staircase. A high wall and heavy wooden door enclosed a spacious yard, an ideal place for the German shepherd dog we acquired to romp with the children and, when we bred her, with her litter of pups.

Also, there we had a wedding. It was the culmination of Maria's venture with our family. Our Chilean helper of seven years and far travels had met and fallen in love with a university student from Yucatan, a devout evangelical believer like herself. After he graduated, I married them in a simple ceremony on our lawn, and soon after we left the country they moved to Yucatan, where he had a good government position. Sadly, he was still in his prime when he died, leaving Maria to go through some lean times with her two daughters. But she and they—with the five children they had between them—have not only survived but also gotten a good education for the children and developed solid character. Maria has turned eighty years old, contented and supported by her own family; although she has never again seen the family she left far south in Antofagasta, Chile. We still keep in touch by e-mail and now through Facebook.

∞∞

When the job I was filling was eliminated, it seemed time to make a change from foreign service. John Jansen, my closest friend in college days, who had become a professor of New Testament at the Presbyterian seminary in Austin, Texas, used his influence to open a door for me to something radically different—teaching elective courses in biblical literature at the University of Texas. Suddenly, I had to be swimming hard to get into the fast-moving stream of biblical scholarship, trying to stay a few strokes ahead of my students. I found it to be exciting and hugely stimulating. Here was a whole new world of questions and challenges that I hadn't even dabbled in while my focus was on the church's mission in Latin America.

For Martha, the change was not as radical, but there was change. In managing our household of eight, she now had no domestic help; although easy access to prepared foods and conveniences of many sorts afforded some compensation. The seminary provided us with a large house and yard, ample space for the children; but it was an old house, drafty in winter and already inhabited by an army of small, curious roaches. My salary was adequate, but not more than adequate for our sizable family, with rare occasions for eating out.

Even so, the children, all but little Larry, were quickly immersed in the Austin school system—only the older ones feeling some pangs of adjustment from what they had loved about our life in Mexico City.

15

Near-Panic on a Frigid Night

2009

The shore had always drawn Martha and me. I've already described the vacation house that we bought at the Jersey shore, when we sold our Bay House in Maryland. A sign of Martha's deepening illness now was a gradual withdrawal, as sea air lost its appeal for her. From Rossmoor we made some trips to our Shore House—never very extended. After our move to Lions Gate, I found it difficult to interest her in going, even for an overnight.

When Sylvia, who was overseas with the United Nations, was back on a visit, that helped. Sylvia enjoyed the shore too, and she knew how much I loved seeing the water. With her encouragement, Martha agreed to spend several days there. One day, we crossed the bridge to Island Beach. There was a cul-de-sac where one could park and follow a zigzag walkway to the top of the dunes, then down a flight of steps into deep sand and the beach. A fresh breeze was blowing, rattling the dry dune grass. In warm sun, there was sand on the boards, inviting bare feet to sink into the deep, softer sand below and go on to the water's edge, as far up as small waves were reaching. Such had been Martha's childhood delight, and we had both loved the sea in all of our years together.

"Don't you want to go down to the beach to feel the sand and see the waves from there?" I urged.

"No, this is enough. You go down. I'll sit here for a while."

There was a bench there, built into the railing. Sylvia stayed with Martha so that I could make a few footprints in the deep sand; but soon, Martha was feeling chilled and wanted to go. The sweep of the Atlantic, the sight and sound of its surf, seemed to mean little to her anymore.

With Sylvia at the Shore House, I had a chance to use the kayak that replaced my former series of sailboats. But when there were just two of us, I had to realize that I couldn't count on making Martha understand where I was going and when I would be back. My nightmare scenario became a picture of me having paddled off toward the bay and Martha going to the dock to peer down the lagoon where I had gone, leaning out too far to see. The water wasn't deep at the edge, but the bottom shelved off to about fifteen feet, and although she had grown up swimming at the beach, who could count on that if she panicked? I still took the kayak out one day, just paddling around nearby, keeping in sight of our dock. After that, it stayed out of water until we sold the house. This was sad for me, but in candor, I had to acknowledge that age was affecting both my joints and balance, making it increasingly hard for me to get in and out of that kayak once I had it afloat.

Our move to Lions Gate brought renewed contacts that were important to us. Pre-eminent among them, and the primary reason for moving to this location, was the proximity to Marilyn, Dale, and their children—Andy, half way through college at Rutgers at the time of our move, and Alex, a rising senior at Eastern Regional High School in Voorhees, and Dale's son Dan, already out of college. Marilyn and Dale's spacious, comfortable house became a second home for us, as well as an inn for other family members when they came to visit. Tom and Janice would drive down, usually at night, from Newton, Massachusetts, spending a day with her parents in their CCRC near Princeton, then a day with us. Larry, June, and their boys, Paul and Will, were in Baltimore, not too far away. Alan and Ron, in Aspen, Colorado, were sometimes in the area; Donna, although far off in California, always managed to be here for special occasions, often with one or two of her three children; and Sylvia, working in Somalia, then Iraq, then South Sudan, took a leave two or three times a year, always staying with us in our apartment. The grandchildren, those out on their own, also visited when they could.

Being back where we once lived, Martha rejoined Trinity Presbyterian Church in Cherry Hill, where she had been organist and director of music forty years earlier. As a Presbyterian minister, I rejoined West Jersey Presbytery, which covers the lowest part of the state. The presbytery meeting at which I was received was convened on the campus of the mental hospital at Ancora, an unusual location, to be sure. It was a January night and extraordinarily cold. On the sprawling campus, I proceeded to what I understood to be the designated parking lot. We were late—as I too often am—and no one was around. I started out with Martha, walking carefully in the early dark, looking for a lighted building and then for an entrance where the meeting might be. It was a relief to find it—to be inside and warm.

The meeting had begun and preliminaries were in progress. The Stated Clerk, who presided over this part of the meeting, had noted our arrival and already had in hand my letter of transfer, enabling me to rejoin this presbytery. He also had taken note of my date of birth. At the appropriate point he announced:

"We are also receiving again a former member, Donald Fletcher, who has moved back to this area. I have to observe that today, January 7th, is his birthday. I can't recall that the presbytery has ever received or re-received, an eighty-nine-year-old minister!"

This netted a ripple of applause as I made my way forward, and the clerk, a personal friend, added, "We welcome Don back, and his charming wife, Martha, who is also present."

After the hour-and-a-half meeting, dealing with a moderate agenda of church business, we lingered for a while. When we left, I didn't notice that it was by a door on a different side of the building from where we had entered. Outside, there seemed to be few light poles and meager illumination, and the bitter cold felt colder. I was very conscious of uneven footing in the dark, holding Martha's arm firmly. This was no place or time for a fall. Most of the others had left, and again, there seemed to be almost no one in sight.

We started for where I thought we had left the car; but when we approached, there was nothing familiar. I tried a different direction—no success. Martha was starting to shake with the cold. Forget about the car— my concern now was to find shelter for her. Most of the buildings were dark. I tried a couple of entries but with no response.

Finally, there was a door with a crack of light, and it wasn't locked. Inside, with immense relief, we met warm air, light, and several friendly people, apparently night staff of the hospital. All I was asking was that I might leave Martha with them while I went to find our car and come back for her. One young woman, a vigorous, outdoor type, wouldn't hear of that.

"You stay in here where it's warm. Describe your car to me, give me the key, I'll find it and bring it back."

"No, I can't do that." I protested.

"Of course you can. You need to stay with your wife." The young woman was already putting on what looked to me like a rather thin coat.

"I at least need to go with you." I insisted. "Martha, you stay here with these good folks; we'll be back soon." I looked into her face. In her eyes there was doubt and uncertainty, but I didn't see fear.

"Where are you going?" she asked.

"Just to get our car. These friends are helping us find our car so we can go home. I'll be back very soon." I gave her a reassuring pat.

My guide, probably understanding these things because of where she was working, was holding the door for me to slip out quickly as she followed. Out in the cold night, I was glad for her hearty confidence. Sure enough, we soon located the car and, to my grateful relief, the cold engine caught after only a couple of turns. It was profoundly good to pull up at that entry, that island of light and warmth, to thank our kind helpers over and over, and to have Martha beside me, shivering again in the cold car, but headed for our apartment home.

16

Later, You'll Be Able to Sing

1960, 1964

We made the move from Mexico City to Austin in the summer of 1960. A few months later, Martha's health faltered—a low fever and feelings of exhaustion. The doctor found that her thyroid was enlarged, which could be dangerous. The growth might be malignant—at that point in medical history he couldn't be sure until after surgery. This all happened quickly, so quickly there wasn't time to be worried. I have a clear image of watching with Martha from the window of her hospital room as all of our six children, clustered on the sidewalk below, were waving to her—no children permitted to visit patients in the hospital. Following fervent prayer and with profound thankfulness, we learned that Martha's tumor was not malignant; the surgery would simply mean that she would be taking a small thyroid supplement daily for the rest of her life. What saddened her was that her hospital roommate, undergoing the same surgery, had the other outcome—malignancy.

In Austin, we entered enthusiastically into the life of University Presbyterian Church—a vigorous congregation with a wealth of human resources and a beautiful, versatile building right across from the main campus. Once more, as seemed to happen wherever we went, a position opened up for Martha and she was soon directing the church's music program. What was different was that here, for the first time, she had the collaboration of a superb organist. Esma Beth Clark could play anything Martha asked for; they formed an effective team and quickly, a deep and lasting friendship. And the church offered out of its large, university-oriented congregation some trained voices and many bright, enthusiastic singers. Under Martha's direction the choir swelled, and children's choirs began to be added.

A high point quite early in our time in Austin was a production of Benjamin Britten's charming musical setting of the medieval mystery play, *Noye's Fludde.* The university's music and drama people who were putting it on turned to Martha to direct the children. In Britten's setting of the play, as skies darken and the deluge approaches the animals appear, flowing up the aisle and crowding onto Noah's ark. But the animals are a children's chorus.

Some talented women of the university community made out of papier-maché a marvelous set of realistically painted, hollow animal heads for the children to wear. Fletcher family members whom Martha incorporated in the chorus were Sylvia (zebra), Tom (giraffe), Marilyn (monkey) and Alan (mouse). When production reached the moment of imminent menace from the deluge, the hall darkened and the orchestral ensemble moved into Britten's storm music. Up the aisle they came, these wonderful animals, streaming and chanting in childish trebles and somewhat more mature sopranos: "Kyrie, Kyrie, Kyrie eleison" (Lord, have mercy). The liturgical refrain became an appeal, made suddenly more powerful when the single voice of a boy soprano, Tom, broke through poignantly, "Kyrie eleison!" The children's part moved harmoniously, blending the pageant together. That was exactly as Martha, with her Westminster training, wished it to be.

Martha loved children, loved singing, and felt that every child could and should share in the joy of it. At University Presbyterian she had plenty of children to work with, as well as eager parental support. But there were, inevitably, some children who had no ear for music, couldn't distinguish pitches, and just droned along in a monotone. If they were interested, Martha gladly worked with them one on one. And when the children's choir sang in church she made them part of the group, even though she wanted the music to be beautiful.

"Just mouth the words," she would tell them. "Make your mouth go, but don't make a sound—for now. Later, you'll be able to sing."

And later they could, in fact, sing—perhaps not a whole melody, but several recognizable tones that harmonized with the rest of the choir.

One child had the extra handicap of being almost deaf, wearing large hearing aids, the best that the technology of the time could offer. Martha took him on as a challenge. She tried every way she could think of to get through the barrier, helping him to recognize and produce sounds on pitch. In the end, she couldn't get this pupil to sing songs; but his parents appreciated warmly that instead of just making noises, he was actually singing his few notes.

The acme of Martha's choral effort at the university church was the performance at Easter of a considerable part of Bach's *St. Matthew Passion*. It was important to accomplish it using only voices and a few instruments drawn from that congregation, with Esma Beth at the organ and the senior pastor as narrator. Martha worked into her home schedule many extra hours of rehearsing the choir and coaching her amateur soloists.

"We're not professionals," she told them at the final rehearsal. "We're not trying to put on a perfect, professional performance. In fact, don't think of this as a performance at all—that wouldn't have been Bach's purpose when he wrote the music. He meant it to be worship, to be a beautiful expression of the passion message offered to God. Let's make everyone who listens feel that when we sing."

When the time came—and after a heartfelt prayer with them, her people, in the choir room—Martha stood, raised her arms and began the solemn, exquisitely paced opening, "Here yet a while…"

She kept her gestures small, which was John Finlay Williamson's way, the way he taught at Westminster. The strength of leadership must come from the bearing, the physique, and the dynamism of the musician standing forward as leader. Hand movements were minimal; direction came via the form and face, the eyes—and Martha must have every eye, none lost in printed music, every eye on her.

I was glad that the church arranged for this performance to be recorded. I had the now old-fashioned LP records in my hands today and was playing them again, a few hours before writing this. It is Easter, almost fifty years later, and I needed that message again.

17

Of Wheelchairs and the Daunting Search for Time Off

2008–2010

Marilyn arranged an outing to Longwood Gardens in the Christmas season, our second Christmas at Lions Gate. Longwood Gardens, thirty miles south of Philadelphia, is an estate originally purchased by Quaker George Peirce from William Penn in 1700, further developed by Pierre du Pont and opened to the public by the du Pont family under the auspices of the Longwood Foundation. The large grounds are beautifully landscaped and endowed with a series of vaulted greenhouses famous for year-round floral displays. Particularly famous—and a huge tourist draw—are the holiday arrangements of poinsettias and all sorts of other festive flowers and Christmas trees in the warm, moist greenhouses, plus half-a-million white lights sparkling on arches and trees all over the grounds. The parking area is set at a discreet distance, which is good for bucolic serenity and, no doubt, for the health of pedestrians, walking the ups and downs of rather long paths over rolling terrain.

For Martha, Dale borrowed a wheelchair from SCUCS (Senior Citizens United Community Services). The wheelchair feature was startling. It had its pleasant side—the ease of rolling along, moving with Martha at a comfortable pace, and securely—no concern about footing nor about whether she would be up to the distances or the grades. In addition, helpful people kept showing consideration to the white-haired lady in the chair, making way for her and holding doors. But the sight of her—my lifelong, once vigorous, independent companion, sitting bundled up *in a wheelchair*, being pushed passively along *in a wheelchair*—that was unnerving. I felt like looking away, like rejecting emphatically that this might be, after all, a regular part of our lives only a little further down the road.

The gardens were beautiful, though—and particularly beautiful was the coming of dusk. We stood a while outside after leaving the bright greenhouses, and a round moon emerging to hang above them put the tiny tree lights in perspective.

❧✧❧

The following winter brought a small incident that reminded me of how careful I needed to be as caregiver-in-chief. We had been over at Marilyn and Dale's for a Sunday-night supper—perhaps a football-game supper. There had been snow, quite a bit of snow, and going home I knew that I needed to take special care. I walked Martha out through the garage, the shortest way to our car parked in the driveway. Dale's snow

blower had done a good job—everything was clear—
and Marilyn watched from the door while I got Martha
seated and we began to move down the driveway. Back
at Lions Gate, maintenance personnel had plowed the
parking areas well. I told Martha that I would pull up
at the foot of the short walkway leading to our entry.
A path had been cleared, with some loose snow piled
at each side.

I stopped the car with what I thought was ample
clearance for Martha to step out on the open walkway.
In effect, after I came around the car, there was clear
space and she got out of the car onto her feet. But we
needed to close the car's wide door for her to proceed
up the walk. I helped Martha move back beside the
car, which meant that I had to step up a slope in the
piled-up snow. There was clearance and the door had
just closed when I slipped, stumbled, and went down,
taking Martha with me as I was all she had to hold
on to.

There we were, side by side, full length in the snow
beside our car. We must have presented a ludicrous
spectacle. I even thought I heard Martha giggle, but I
was too chagrined and too eager for recovery to notice
that. I struggled to my feet as quickly as I could, then
warily and with relief, managed to help Martha get to
hers, joining in brushing snow from her bulky coat.
A furtive look around and toward the lighted entry
reassured me that no one had watched our tumble.

With solicitous care, I guided my wife up the short
walk to that welcoming door and into the warmth of
the foyer, down the long corridor to the elevator and,

at last, to our own familiar apartment. She offered no comment, then or afterward, about what had happened. And, as if we were a pair of teenagers and they were our parents, I said nothing about the misadventure to our daughter and son-in-law. Well aware that I was not as young, strong, and secure as I wanted to feel—nor, likely, as capable of caring for Martha in all situations, I chose to let the incident go by as a humorous happening that could have been more—a reminder of how careful I needed to be.

∞ ∞

Our energetic program director at Lions Gate organized, one morning a week, a small group of residents with some memory impairment. Known simply as the Club, the group engaged in a variety of activities designed to challenge and stimulate the brain. I took Martha, staying with her at first and joining in. Then, as an off-shoot, a smaller caregivers support group emerged, and we were given an excellently qualified, young social worker with special training to be our leader. For several of us, this group became—and has continued to be—a high point of our week.

Through the group, I was encouraged to look outside for a place where I might leave Martha with other seniors for several hours at a time—a place offering structured activity adapted to the needs of dementia clients, accomplishing what the Lions Gate club was trying to accomplish, but having more people, more resources, and more time. I found that there was such a facility, called Senior Care, very near us. I went to visit it and proceeded to enroll Martha.

Things seemed promising at first. Martha would have congenial surroundings, be well taken care of and usefully engaged for several hours, three days a week; and I could get valuable time off to refresh my body and mind.

The promising beginning didn't last. Martha began to resist going to Senior Care; then the resistance notched up to flat refusal. Something else had to be found.

Many residents of Lions Gate used the services of home-health aides. I went to our staff nurse for advice and she spread out on her desk eight or ten brochures of agencies providing such service. "Take your pick," she said, plainly intending not to recommend one above another. I selected four brochures to take home for study and ended up choosing an agency that was among the earliest; it had now spread through several states, seemed well-organized and competitively priced and, intriguingly, had been founded by the wife of a Presbyterian minister. The agency, which has a branch office in a town very nearby, sent a representative to visit. In short order, Martha was enrolled, a schedule arranged, and we were expecting our first helper. She (most of the aides are women) would come for four hours, two mornings a week. This was in January, 2010.

Our monthly fee at Lions Gate was taking up two-thirds of our income that came almost entirely from my church pension, our two state pensions for our years as public school teachers, and social security. When we took out, further, the ten percent of gross income that we divided among causes that we chose to support, the margin left for car, health insurance, and other expenses was not large. But adequate care for Martha must be primary, and the help of home- health aides now seemed to be part of it. We had some reserves from the sale of our house at the shore and other sources. I would begin to draw on these as necessary—and with Alzheimer's encroaching, such necessity was certain to increase.

18

To Mississippi;
to Deter Violence

1964, 1965

O ur years in Austin, the first half of the 1960's decade, were a time of ferment. The Cold War Space Race was on, with the USSR leading. Yuri Gagarin made his orbit, the first human in space, in the spring of 1961. I remember at an outdoor swim club straining my eyes to glimpse a bright speck that was supposed to be visible in the afternoon sky, the latest Russian sputnik passing over. Much closer at hand, the civil rights struggle was working into the national consciousness. In the summer of 1964, the Freedom Summer, hundreds of young people from northern states poured into the Deep South to support a voter registration drive for black citizens. They met some fierce, fanatical resistance. It was the summer that saw the murders of three young men, Cheney, Schwerner, and Goodman—civil rights activists, one black, two white—in Mississippi.

One call that went out to help the civil rights effort was for the Hattiesburg Ministers Project. Hattiesburg, Mississippi, was a focal point of the voter registration drive.

"Martha, I think I ought to take part in this Hattiesburg project," I proposed.

"You? What would you do?"

"The call is for ministers just to be there, to go along with the young people who are helping black citizens register to vote. They aren't to take part directly—just be present as a deterrent to violence."

"I don't know. This family needs you here. The children need you and I need you. Isn't Mississippi where those three young men were killed?"

"It is, but there are a lot of volunteers still working there. This would be a way to help to give them support and have a hand in the most important thing happening in this country right now."

Reluctantly, Martha agreed. "If that's what you feel you must do, you do it. But please, be careful, and don't be away too long. It gets hard when you're not here."

I signed on for a week in Hattiesburg. The civil rights struggle was a seething pot. For me, the effect of the experience was profound—from the first evening when, after some grueling hours of briefing, we stood in a circle with our leaders; white and black, locked arms, and sang a song I was hearing for the first time, "We Shall Overcome". I found myself adopting, in a single day, a new perspective. Quartered in a firehouse in the heart of the black district of Hattiesburg, I quickly got to feeling safe only when I was in that part of the city— when all the faces in the neighborhood were black. Out in the community, with its mixture of white and black, there was always uneasiness; and the sight of a white sheriff or policeman, even at a distance, meant a sudden tightening of the gut.

One evening a group of us was gathered in the home of a maverick University of Southern Mississippi professor who supported the civil rights movement. Abruptly he broke off conversation, asking a young black woman to move. He had realized that she was sitting opposite the front doorway that afforded a clear shot from the shrubbery outside. Another day, my assignment— because I was teaching at the University of Texas—was to wander around the university campus, just to chat with students and perhaps faculty members, with an eye toward promoting understanding of our group's peaceful and positive intention for the community. I succeeded in getting a favorable hearing from a few students, but in a short while I was summoned by one of the deans and ordered off campus, under threat of action by the campus police. When some of us tried to attend service in a Hattiesburg Presbyterian church, we were told bluntly by church officers standing in the door that we were not welcome. After my stay in Mississippi it was natural enough, although it surprised me, that I felt a surge of relief when the bus came to the state line and we were crossing into Louisiana.

∞·∞

Our happy and productive years in Austin came to an end in 1965, when I again found myself without a job. Independent support from three church denominations, which had enabled me to teach at the university, collapsed.

Yet, Martha's work at University Church was thriving. The people there were devoted to her and eager to keep moving on to better things. Jane, wife of the seminary president, was one of Martha's most loyal supporters. She had a beautiful voice, and Martha occasionally gave her solo parts; she taught Jane's children piano, as well. It seemed likely that Jane was the motivating force when David, her husband, came one evening to talk and to offer me a job. The seminary's librarian was leaving; I could get a little preparation and step into that position. In response to my query, though, David made it clear that I would do no teaching; the teaching faculty was complete.

He seemed surprised and disappointed when, after due thanks and appreciation, I declined the offer. Work in the library, with no prospect of teaching? No, that could not be for me. David remarked later, "You might at least have said you'd like a day or two to think it over."

What opened up for me was an opportunity at Stillman College, a predominantly black Presbyterian college in Tuscaloosa, Alabama. There I could teach English and chair the English Department and the Division of Humanities, using directly for the first time the PhD in English that I had completed at Princeton some fifteen years earlier. So, we left Austin. Martha's choir at University Presbyterian, in their sad farewell, gave her a beautiful, sterling silver table service for twelve (still treasured in its felt-lined chest in our closet). We were leaving behind dear friends—Esma Beth and her husband, Jimmy, in particular—with whom we would stay in touch and visit over many years. And we were leaving Donna, who was about to spend her first year at the University of Texas.

19

Drastic Consequences
of a Fall

2010

Martha and I had been living at Lions Gate for almost three years when it happened. The situation was so simple and natural—the event, catastrophic. I had made an appointment for Martha to have a permanent at a small hair salon where she had known Jean (not her actual name), the proprietor, from fourteen years earlier when we lived in the area. Pulling up in front of the shop on this pleasant day, I helped Martha out of the car and walked her in, holding her arm.

"Here she is, Jean."

Jean, always kind and attentive, came to meet us. We were exchanging the usual sort of pleasantries, including my remarking on this being the day after our wedding anniversary, May 19, our sixty-eighth. Martha, meanwhile, was not listening, distracted by other things in the room. I arranged to come back in an hour and a half and was preparing to leave.

What I hadn't noticed, and neither had Jean, was that Martha had moved around behind her. Saying goodbye, Jean turned, taking a step back, and bumped

Martha. It was only a slight bump, but too much for Martha's uncertain balance. She went down, brushing against one of the salon's swivel chairs that somewhat broke her fall.

Aghast, we bent over her. She was stretched full length, startled, but seemed unhurt. "Thank God," Jean said, "nothing seems to be broken."

We helped Martha sit up and that was when the pain started. She cried out, and wouldn't move any more. Jean had her helper call 911.

The emergency people agreed that it looked like a hip fracture. They brought in their gurney, but Martha screamed at any change of position. That was when they produced a wonderful, hinged device with flat plates that slid under Martha just as she was, half-sitting, and let them lift her onto the gurney and into the ambulance with no further movement. At the hospital the diagnosis was confirmed. This was Thursday. Surgery could be scheduled for Friday evening.

I had a problem. Two weeks earlier, with Marilyn looking after her mother, I had made an overnight trip to Duarte, just outside Los Angeles, to see my brother, Arch, who was very ill. Four days later Arch died. There was to be a memorial service on Saturday, May 22, and I would have a part in it. I had my ticket to fly to the West Coast again on Friday—but that was now the day of Martha's surgery. Marilyn urged me to go; my trip was too important to be canceled. She would stay with Martha and see her through the surgery, and my return flight would get me back on Sunday.

At the hospital Friday evening Marilyn was doing her part. She held Martha's hand, talking reassuringly, until the gurney was wheeled through the door of the operating suite; then she sat down in the now-empty waiting room for a solitary vigil—Friday evening and all very quiet. But only a moment later the corridor door opened and the tall surgeon was coming through. Seeing Marilyn, he stopped for a brisk, friendly word.

"Your mother will be fine. This is a surgery that we do all the time. It takes a couple of hours, maybe three, and of course she'll be completely out of it after that. Why don't you just go along? I'll call you at home when it's finished, and you can come see your mother in the morning."

Marilyn hesitated, but she could see the sense in the doctor's advice. As she found, even in the morning Martha was hardly aware. It was only by the second morning, Sunday, when I saw her that she was beginning to be more awake. We had drawn an excellent surgeon, one of the best, and the wizardry of hip replacement is now such that on that second day after the operation Martha was able to stand and put full weight on her mended hip with no evident pain. If only the rest of recovery could have been that easy!

Rather, what we began to realize was that the trauma of the accident and subsequent surgery and hospitalization had pushed Martha's Alzheimer's far down the road. The creeping shadow of eclipse had suddenly darkened. Much had been lost in the half-second of that fall and its aftermath. When I consulted him about it, our family doctor confirmed that the trauma related to an accident of this sort usually has a markedly negative effect on the condition of an Alzheimer's patient.

When I was back, Martha didn't want me out of her sight. I stayed in her room and slept that night in the armchair, although for the next couple of nights the children convinced me that I should go home. Tom came down from Boston, and was there to help when Martha left the hospital. Larry, Donna, and daughter Jessica all were on hand for part or all of the following weekend that included Memorial Day.

∽∾

From the hospital, we moved Martha to Genesis, a rehabilitation facility three or four miles from Lions Gate. Why not bring her directly to Lions Gate that has excellent accommodation in its skilled nursing facility? Because Lions Gate did not have a contract with our insurance company that would cover physical therapy as part of rehabilitation, and Genesis did.

The people at Genesis were helpful, particularly those in the therapy department, but much had changed. Martha seemed sluggish, as if some effect of the anesthesia were carrying over. She slept a lot. When the nurse's aides could get her up, it had to be to a wheelchair. She seemed unable to walk and had developed a deep, rattling cough that was disconcerting.

I came to know the drive to Genesis very well, and the choice of routes one could take. A time or two, I ate Martha's meal for her, because she had little appetite.

And there was scant communication. She said, or tried to say, a few words from time to time, but they were often indistinct and disconnected. She seemed aware and would smile at the staff people who came into the room or at her roommate's visitors, but did little more. I couldn't tell how much of what I said to her was understood. And that rattling cough held on.

The speech therapist proposed, and the doctor concurred, that Martha should have a glottal test at a hospital where they had this facility. Again, as when she was brought to Genesis, I watched while she was rolled in her wheelchair onto the lift, raised and eased into the medical transport bus; then I sat where I could reach to hold her hand while the bus bumped along its way.

The glottal test showed that swallowing was, in fact, the problem. When Martha swallowed, the epiglottis was not closing off tightly, letting some liquid leak into her lungs. All liquids should be thickened and she should have only puréed food. In effect, with this change the cough cleared up in a couple of days, but the puréed diet and thickened liquids had to be continued.

The physical therapy room at Genesis became a place where I felt a little brightness. The therapists seemed genuinely, not just professionally, hopeful and upbeat. They soon had Martha standing, then taking a few faltering steps with a walker, the wheelchair always right behind if she needed it. I would look forward to these sessions, feeling real disappointment when the room was closed and our time there had to be missed.

At the noon meal hour after a few days, I could take Martha to the dining room. She had a place at a table of four. I could pull up a chair to sit and feed her, becoming acquainted with her tablemates in their various stages of rationality. For some days an unkempt, bearded man sat alone at one side of the large room, erupting in snatches of songs or in loud demands for attention. I picked up no clue as to his identity or history, or who had brought him to the facility, but we all were relieved when he stopped appearing. Martha's tablemates were quiet. At some other tables there would be bursts of strident voices and clashing of dishes and flatware, and we had a busman who seemed to enjoy clearing tables with maximum clatter while pushing a trash cart with inexplicably screeching wheels.

The best times I had with Martha were intervals in the garden. Some days, if the weather was pleasant, I could roll her out to an enclosed area where there were tables, benches, and garden chairs under a few trees. Some staff would take their breaks there, and an occasional patient might appear, but there was ample space. I could sit and read a few pages, or just watch some sparrows foraging for crumbs under a table, listen to twittering in the branches above, and feel the warmth and peace. Martha might look around, not appearing really interested in anything, or would simply doze. Some days she seemed content, and we could just be together there. Other days, she became agitated after a little, wanting to go in. Then we had to move.

It was early in the two weeks at Genesis that Donna and Jessica came and on another day, Larry. The family was loyally supporting me as much as Martha—perhaps

I wasn't admitting how I needed that support. They learned the Genesis routine and we sat and talked, dragging garden chairs together on paving blocks dappled by the overhanging tree.

20

Her Own *Noye's Fludde*

1967, 1971

We were on the move again. I'd accepted a position as a secretary for continuing education with the Presbyterian Board of Christian Education in Philadelphia. It had seemed time to leave Stillman College in Tuscaloosa. The college had installed a black president, the first in its history. I saw an opportunity to open the way for a black colleague to chair the English Department, while we returned to familiar ground in the Philadelphia area. In Cherry Hill, New Jersey, Martha and I found a large-enough home that we could afford with an easy commute to my office in the city.

The surprise came while we were at Mo-Ranch, a Presbyterian conference center in Texas, sharing in a vacation/youth conference before our move. There was a long distance call for Martha from the organizing pastor of Trinity Presbyterian Church in Cherry Hill, New Jersey. The fast-growing congregation was in need of an organist/director of music. Would she be interested?

"Well, yes, of course...but how?"

Pastor Ed's reply went something like this: "I know. You're all the way down there in Texas; but I know that you are moving to this area, and your reputation has gotten here ahead of you."

Martha was thrilled at the prospect, while we both were left wondering how Ed had gotten his information. My guess was that he had somewhere been in touch with the senior pastor at University Presbyterian in Austin. That could at least explain the *reputation* part.

The trip back east amounted to a family caravan with a distinctly Toonerville Trolley appearance. We had our station wagon with Martha and me and the four younger children, and a vacation camper behind. There was also a small, much-used car we'd gotten for Donna in college. She was driving it with Sylvia for company and, behind all that, my outboard boat on its trailer. A memorable moment came at our entrance to Baltimore, when signs warned that the propane tank on our camper couldn't go through the harbor tunnel. I quickly took an exit, only to sit and watch helplessly as Donna's little car and the boat—too far back to have noticed our turn off—went serenely on above us. There were no cell phones, then, to alert Donna and Sylvia to our turn off, nor to help us finally get together on the other side of Baltimore. The sensation of that moment stayed with me, a symbol of how the children were beginning to grow up and move on—our family circle drawing in.

꩜꩜꩜

Trinity Presbyterian Church became a center of our new life. Cherry Hill was, quintessentially, a suburban residential community. My job involved frequent travel; Martha had the major role in homemaking and family life, with the four younger children soon immersed in the competitive environment of Cherry Hill's excellent school system. Trinity Church was expanding along with the vibrant community. The presbytery's foresight in planting its new church had included acquisition of a strategically-located site and erection of a sanctuary with a tall spire and arresting façade. By the time we were settled, Pastor Ed had left, but his young associate, installed as senior pastor, moved ahead with adding Martha to the team.

Before long, with her characteristic energy and commitment to her ideal of music at the heart of the church in full-voiced expression of faith in God, Martha was adding choirs, recruiting people at all levels. There came to be two adult choirs—one for each Sunday morning service—and a range of children and youth choirs from the small, irresistible cherubs up to senior high. For some years, Trinity operated schools of faith—midweek evening events that brought what seemed like hordes of school children and some parents to the church for a simple supper, followed by classes of Christian instruction, alternating with choir rehearsals. The scene could appear chaotic, bursting with life, but Martha held firm in the thick of it.

This was also a time when the use of English handbells was spreading among American congregations. Martha seized on the challenge, organizing a group of mainly younger women who raised money to buy and later expand a set of the bells.

They worked enthusiastically, learning the techniques as Martha was learning ahead of them, some mothers among them bringing their small children and improvising childcare. And the congregation responded with pleasure to the addition the handbell music made to worship.

One signal musical event of Martha's tenure at Trinity Church was her production of Britten's *Noye's Fludde.* She had enjoyed her share in the performance of the work in Austin by the University of Texas. Now she had the resources to plan and direct her own production. The animal heads for the children's choir were only two-dimensional—not like the hollow papier-mâché creations of the ladies in Austin—but they still made for a gripping, colorful procession when the children poured up the central aisle chanting their "Kyrie eleison". And the ark, I thought, outdid the Austin production.

That was because my share was designing and supervising the construction of it. I wanted it to suggest a medieval sailing ship, in keeping with the medieval mystery play that Britten set to music. The ship was in several sections—light wooden frames covered with cloth, on which some of the women painted realistic timbers and heraldic insignia. Above the ship, a tall mast with spar and square sail almost filled the chancel. When the moment of the storm scene came, with sanctuary darkened and a projected light from the rear balcony flickering like lightning, the mast and billowing sail were made to sway on their stays, and the

whole chancel seemed to heave and rock to the cadence
of the navy hymn:

> Eternal Father, strong to save,
> Whose arm doth bind the restless wave,
> ...
> O hear us when we cry to Thee
> For those in peril on the sea.

21

So We'll Talk No More, My Love

2010

After fourteen days, we moved Martha from Genesis to Lions Gate's skilled nursing facility. Tom was again on hand to help with the move. At Genesis, the insurance would begin to require a sizable daily co-pay; at Lions Gate, without insurance we could use some of Martha's *bank days*—up to ninety days in assisted living or skilled nursing without additional charge—as provided in our original contract. We would have to pay personally for therapy, but that should still cost less than the co-pay at Genesis; and a major plus would be the ease with which I could walk from our apartment, through a series of corridors and protected doors, right to Martha's room at any time.

The skilled-nursing scene at Lions Gate was different—psychologically, emotionally, as well as in simple, structural ways. Genesis had been more like a hospital, with patient rooms lined up along corridors, although there was the therapy room and the timber-ceilinged dining room that served also for social activities. At Lions Gate, Martha's room was part of a cluster, opening on a sitting room with a large television.

Down a short corridor was the principal common room, with the nurse's station at one side. Most of the patients gathered there by walker or wheelchair, the majority in various stages of dementia. The program director did effective service, organizing simple games and activities that some could share—but even these now proved to be beyond what Martha could do. When I came by after dinner, I might find her wheelchair drawn up with others to the table for Bingo. She could be watching, distracted by the movement and voices, but not participating.

The pattern I adopted was to be with Martha in the afternoon and wheel her to the dining room when the dinner call came, which was rather early. I would set her at an assigned place and draw up a chair beside her. Martha's puréed food would eventually arrive—a dinner plate with small mounds that had started out as chicken, peas and carrots, baked potato, or whatever was on the menu that day. The mounds were identical in texture, distinguishable only by pale shades of color. My part was to help Martha, who sometimes made some effort to manage a spoon, and to encourage her to keep eating. Generally, her appetite seemed better than mine would have been, contemplating those nondescript mounds on the plate.

She had two tablemates. One was a woman who was very deaf and almost blind. She needed special food that she called for loudly and insistently; although we found that she responded gratefully to a gesture of kind concern. The other tablemate was a Polish grandfather attended by a private aide, a pleasant Hispanic woman, who was adroit at handling his stubbornness and occasional outbursts. He too was on the puréed diet, which she could get him to eat in spite of his dogged resistance.

When Martha was finished, I would leave her in the common room and go back to the independent-living section of Lions Gate, to have dinner in the main dining rooms before returning to her. It was on one of those long June evenings as I sat with her in the quiet of her room, waiting for dark and for the nurse's aide to come and prepare her for the night, that I began to write the poem "Evening". Alzheimer's eclipsing shadow was closing off almost all communication. The opening of Byron's lyric, "So we'll go no more a-roving/ by the light of the moon," came into my mind and lines began to form. Memory brought back a summer evening at our Bay House on the upper Chesapeake, and an evening scene, much earlier, of Martha practicing at the organ in an empty church. The pain and struggle and my despondence over so much lost since Martha's fall poured into my lines then, and later on as I finished them. They are at the front of the book, and I put them here again.

> So we'll talk no more, my love,
> The moon is almost down.
> Few words are left; none to express
> What we have shared of loveliness,
> Of swallows skimming grass at dusk,
> And firefly sparks among the trees,
> Of organ music in a shadowy nave,
> One soft light only on your face and hands

And whiteness of the keys.
In our silence, now, I hold you, warm and dear
As always—hold you here, and yet not here—
Your smile flickering on the edge of time,
As you move deeper into the not-time
And I reach you less and less. Love, it's still you,
Making the passage gently, by degrees.
I'll make it, too, sometime—we still count
      time—
And we will talk again; or need no words
For perfect sharing—in God's harmony.

22

Life Breaking into Life

1968, 1973

The spring after our move back to New Jersey, 1968, brought around the 25th reunions of our graduating classes—Martha's from Westminster Choir College and mine from Princeton Seminary. We went back, enjoying scenes at Westminster and around Princeton town that evoked memories of our early relationship. They prompted from me these lines:

> And so, my love, what now? We have been back
> To Princeton in the spring, where once, spring
>   was
> A pain in joy, tumultuous, a cry
> Of life-and-love desire that soundlessly
> Broke from our parted lips within the shade
> Of new-leafed branches, white moon dappled.
>   Love,
> That spring is gone, and I'll not buy it back,
> If you won't—not for what the years have cost
> That we have shared, the good and bitter years.
> "Ripeness is all." It's hard to ripen well
> Without the frost and worm and rot. My love,
> I'll take such mellow sweetness as you are,
> And leave the fragile fragrance of that spring
> To blow its faint regret from long ago.

CRCD

Everything about our house had to be right, outside and inside. Larry was even fixing a hinge and painting the gate of the picket fence to our backyard. Donna was getting married. She had met Eric out in Kansas City. He had come once for a visit—a sort of traditional asking the parents for their daughter's hand—as if we had anything to say about that. We liked him immediately and heartily approved Donna's choice. Her further choice was to be married at home—no church wedding, no elaborate reception, just the family and a very few friends. Eric's mother would come from Washington State; he was an only child and his father had died.

Martha took everything in hand. A special touch was that Donna wanted to wear her mother's wedding dress, the sculpted white satin that Della Bradway helped select thirty-one years before. Della would be there and Martha's sister and brother and their spouses; her father was gone. We borrowed folding chairs from the church, saving a space by the piano at the far end of the living room. Alan, already an accomplished pianist, was commissioned to play—Martha needed to be free after all the preparations to enter quietly into her daughter's wedding. When the moment approached, she took her place in the first row. I stood in my pulpit robe at the foot of the stairs, and our first-born came down, radiant as her mother had been, although so different in her person and in this place and time.

After the service, the more senior family members sat in the screened-in back porch, while others filled the dining room and spilled over outside in the October sunshine for a wedding luncheon. Martha had prepared it herself, all but a turkey that a friend insisted on contributing. And in her usual, cheerfully diplomatic way, Martha was seeing to it that things were happening when and how they had been planned.

∽∾

My job in Philadelphia included many flights around the country. Always, the emotional magnet in Cherry Hill was pulling me toward home. At the time, I was trying my hand poetically at the austerely simple, three-line haiku form. From one flight, looking down on a snowy February landscape, came this piece:

> Snowy hills and mist
> of a winter evening; I
> return to my love.

An autumn evening a couple of years later brought this one:

> Geese on evening sky
> asking a passing question
> of place, time, and home.

And there were these lines "To Martha" from about this time:

Peace, my love; I wish you peace today.
I have at other times wished other things,
Beauty and warmth, long time to work and pray,
Love growing rich and deep, happiness that
     sings,
Life breaking into life; but for today
I wish you peace.

In the bustle of life I was perhaps feeling—as I have often felt—how necessary it is to keep open a way to an inner sanctum of serenity.

23

I Want To Go Home

2010

Physical therapy had to be strategic, after Martha's fall and subsequent surgery. It seemed that we had made a good start at Genesis, and I was anticipating a more sustained effort in the therapy room at Lions Gate. I followed as an aide rolled Martha down in her wheelchair. When her turn came, one of the therapists, analyzing her case, crouched beside her and began his friendly instructions. He asked her to try extending her right leg, but she didn't move. Plainly, she didn't understand. He tried something different. Putting her knees together and holding lightly on each side, he told her to try to separate them by pushing against his hands. She looked at him, but made no effort. For several minutes more, the therapist asked Martha to make a variety of movements, even coaching the movements with his hands; however, there was no response.

"Your wife," he said to me, "is not a candidate for therapy, because she can't follow instructions."

They did get her to her feet to take a few steps with a walker, as I told them that she had done at Genesis. Determined to try to make progress, I kept her coming back for several days in spite of the therapist's negative assessment. Then I learned that Martha's insurance would pay for at-home therapy and I found Jim, a therapist who offered that service.

Now we had a new pattern. Three days a week, I rolled Martha through the secure doors and long corridors to our apartment. Just to have her there, even briefly, was a tonic. Then Jim would appear for three quarters of an hour of personal attention in that familiar, peaceful environment. His friendly, easygoing style was effective. He focused entirely on standing and walking, on moving around the apartment, then out in the corridor. In time, at my suggestion, we took Martha in her chair to our parked car, and Jim showed me the moves he helped her make to get from the chair into the car. Now we could have more freedom. Gaining confidence, I could put Martha in the car, leave the wheelchair inside the entry to our building, then drive over to Marilyn and Dale's or any short distance.

The question was how soon I could have Martha at home in our apartment. The final word could come only from the doctor responsible for patients in skilled nursing, and she proved hard to reach. My go-between was the head nurse, who was sympathetic. She could understand how anxious I was, but I should understand their responsibility to be sure that Martha's needs would be met, and the care I would provide was complete enough, that she wouldn't very shortly be requiring re-admission to their facility. The nurse assured me that this happened all too often.

I promised that I would have aides to help care for Martha, and the doctor signed her release. What a liberating experience to go to Martha's room, pick up the bag containing her last items of clothing and personal care, then wheel her through the common room, saying goodbye to staff and fellow patients! Did she recognize or know any of them? It didn't matter. Her warm smile and wave were enough, and these she had for everyone. So, after the elevators, the doors, the succession of corridors and common rooms, we were finally at our own door. I had Martha at home—now it would be up to me.

∞∞

The puréed diet and thickened liquids had to continue. Our pattern came to be that I would take Martha in her wheelchair to the skilled nursing kitchen in late afternoon to pick up her dinner. Back at the apartment, I would roll her up to our table and help her with the puréed fare that was her meal. Then our aide would appear at six o'clock, and I would be free to go to the dining room, joining friends at one table or another and enjoying the pause.

When I returned to the apartment at eight, the aide would have Martha tucked in bed for the night. It was summer and the evenings were long, but generally Martha was soon asleep. One blessing for us in coping with her illness is that, having always been a sound sleeper, she mostly has continued so. She may find a comfortable position after getting in bed, and ten or even twelve hours later she hasn't moved. In these months after her accident she sometimes concerned me by being in bed as long as sixteen hours before being persuaded to get up.

◯◯◯◯

The therapy sessions with Jim ended, but I kept on determinedly with the effort, seconded by our aides. Part of the agreement when Martha was discharged from skilled nursing was that I would have an aide every morning to assist with bathing, dressing, and breakfast, in addition to the aide who came in the evening. I set the hours at 9:00 a.m. to 1:00 p.m., giving me the morning free for occasional meetings or other activities and for reading, working on writing projects, or swimming a routine quarter mile in the pool.

At breakfast, the important and unvarying element came to be hot instant oatmeal. Sylvia had an acquaintance whose mother had suffered from Alzheimer's, and who pointed her to an article that Dr. Mary Newport had published in the St. Petersburg Times on July 22, 2008. Dr. Newport described her experience with coconut oil in treating her husband's early-onset Alzheimer's. She had come to think that ketone bodies produced by the liver from coconut oil might help with the faltering communication in the brain. When Steve, her husband, began taking about two tablespoons of extra-virgin coconut oil daily, he experienced an almost immediate, remarkable improvement, as demonstrated in two drawings of a clock face that he made. One showed only some random, uneven circles—what he was able to remember and sketch before the coconut oil regimen; the other, a single larger circle with spoke-like lines and some numbers, drawn two weeks after beginning it.

Coconut oil seemed simple enough to try. I found it to be light, with little taste, pleasant enough when blended into the oatmeal prepared in the microwave. We both began to use it, finding a good source and price on the internet. Has it proved to be a wonder drug? No. But I am ready to believe that it has been a significant factor in slowing Martha's decline, even in registering a considerable return—both physical and cognitive—toward where she was before her accident.

❦

After therapist Jim had shown Martha how she could move from her wheelchair to the front seat of our car, we were able to resume a particular pleasure, occasional dinner visits in Marilyn and Dale's home. At first, Dale arranged for a wheelchair at their end, in which Martha could manage the one step up at their front door; but we soon realized that she could walk the shorter route through the garage with just the support of a firm arm. In professional football, Marilyn and Dale are Philadelphia Eagles fans. Now we could again go to their house on Sunday evening for a TV-tray supper and the game that the big-screen TV had been recording if the game had already started. Martha seemed to enjoy the company and the festive mood, even if she didn't follow the action on the screen. Once in a while she would get restless, wanting to *go home*, but generally could be persuaded to stay, unless it was a West Coast late-finishing game.

∞∞

Those who have coped with Alzheimer's or other severe dementia know how obsessive the word *home*— and the idea of it—can become. Our apartment is of moderate size—two bedrooms (we use the smaller as a den), two baths, a dining/living room, and a kitchen. This is one of the smaller homes Martha and I have shared. According to my count, it is our twenty-sixth home of one sort or another—borrowed, rented, or owned—over the course of our marriage. Furnishing it entirely with familiar objects from previous homes, I wanted it to feel familiar, as well as snug and secure. But inevitably, the plea has come from Martha at times, "I want to go home."

"But you are home," I answer. "See—all these familiar things; they're what we've had, where we've been. We cleared out and sold the house in Rossmoor—that's gone. Now we're here. This is our home, and it's a good place to be. We have everything we need. We have kind friends to help us and to be with at dinner; and we have Marilyn and her family nearby. It's all good, and it's home."

Such talk seldom succeeds with Martha. Logic— an appeal to reason—has little force with Alzheimer's. Sometimes it just seems to make her angry. Sometimes there are tears, real anguish that is deeply distressing for me. The solution may be to find some distraction, something to deflect the focus, or else just to show affection, trying to convey understanding and reassurance. On the positive side, insistently and in every way that I can, I keep up with the propaganda: apartment 248, the door with the white plate and the little sailboat and big letters, The Fletchers—this is home, our comfortable and secure little home. We have a round, ceramic white plaque with sailboat and name that Larry and June gave us years ago for the Bay House on the Chesapeake; now it stands in a holder on the ledge outside our door, a landmark for our apartment.

In one recent occurrence of the home syndrome we happened to be standing in the short hallway of our apartment. Martha glanced at several of the family pictures on the wall, and abruptly and forcefully came the declaration, "I want to go home." *Home*, it would appear, might be any pulse of memory, any half-formed connection with better times in better places than she is feeling now. And *home*, I believe, may also represent some sense of the capacity, the physical and mental abilities, that were part of those better times and have largely been lost. Perhaps Martha needs and wants that comfort; that sense of capacity and accomplishment that is gone. She needs somehow to find her way back—needs me to take her (surely, I can take her) back to that lost place and time—back to her and our home.

We sat later that afternoon on the sofa that looks out the living room windows toward the woods and driveways and through trees, when leaves are gone, to the traffic moving on Laurel Oak Road. Martha began to see, again, something I couldn't see—something that agitated her. She started to get up.

"Come on…go…let's go. I want to go home."

Taking her hand, wanting her to stay there with me, I protested to her, "This is home, right here. We're home."

"Don't say that! Don't keep saying that!"

"But it is. There's nothing out there. This is home, our home, yours—"

Suddenly she flared out, turning on me fiercely, her face furious, "I hate you! Don't tell me! I hate you!"

Words were useless; I held them back—just let her stand and go toward the window, while I followed to stand behind her. A minute or two passed, then she turned and sat down again. She put her hand on mine. She seemed not to remember what she had said or why she said it. And after dinner, as we started *home*, walking with her walker, she squeezed my arm with hers and said, "I love you."

24

The Beans Are Magic

1974, 1984

For a third time in my career, the job I was doing was eliminated, prompting me to take a new direction. Nationally, the Presbyterian Church (USA) was shrinking and revenues were down. One decision was to reduce positions and draw the major church agencies together in New York, including the Board of Christian Education that had been in Philadelphia.

With my position scrubbed, I thought I'd like to return to college teaching; but the economy was weak, enrollments were down, and the smaller liberal arts colleges—my potential job market—were letting people go, not hiring. I did have one good offer from a church-related college in North Dakota. After visiting the school, I would have taken the job; but when I got back, Martha and the two boys still at home protested, "North Dakota? That's too far!"

I had run for the Cherry Hill school board—my sole experience campaigning for an elected public position— and was finishing my first term. The superintendent of the district, now a trusted friend, knew my situation. "Have you considered high school teaching?" he asked.

"No, I haven't; but at this point I'm ready to consider anything."

Martha found the idea of public school teaching appealing. Within a couple of weeks, we were launched together on a hectic summer of intensive courses at Glassboro State College (now Rowan University) to earn certification, she in music and I in English. It was a hot summer, and the hours were many that we had to juggle to get all the requirements squeezed in, but we managed. The Cherry Hill school district was booming, new hires being made; but in English, I was on a low rung of the ladder with about twelve ahead of me. The weeks kept passing and progress up the ladder was uncertain; thus, a great relief when in mid-August, with school opening not that far away, word came that I had a place in the English Department at Cherry Hill High School West.

Martha's Cherry Hill application was less successful—music is a specialty that school districts add after all the basics are covered. Fortunately, there was a friend whose area of school supervision included Brooklawn, a blue-collar neighborhood some miles south of Cherry Hill. Gerry, the friend, knew and admired Martha's combination of ability and commitment and got her a contract to teach elementary school music in Brooklawn.

By early spring of that first school year, Martha had met many parents and gotten a feel for Brooklawn. She was always interested in people—the children she was given to work with and the homes they came from. The next time she talked with Gerry, her sponsor and supervisor, she had a proposal. The dialogue went something like this:

"You know, Gerry, I've heard in some school districts how they try to put on a popular Broadway musical or parts of it, even with elementary school kids."

Gerry was a vigorous person. She wore her frankly-graying hair short, which seemed to fit her personality. She was quick to answer, "Yes, and I don't like it. These kids grow up soon enough; why push it? But I don't imagine you were going to suggest putting on *South Pacific* in Brooklawn."

Martha joined briefly in the laugh. "No, not quite. But I want the children to have a chance to do something together, something creative and even beautiful that all who want to can have a part in."

"That's great, my dear. God knows a lot of these kids don't have much beauty in their lives—least of all, artistic beauty. So, where do you find the kind of music you're talking about?"

"I'm going to write it. I was thinking about children's stories, stories we all heard when we were little that could still say something to these kids. I came up with Jack and the Beanstalk."

"Jack and the Beanstalk. Hmmm....A Beanstalk Grows in Brooklawn—sorry, I'm not making fun. I like the idea."

That was enough approval for Martha; she ran with it. I wasn't taken into her creative process. Quite alone, she put together a script and laid out scenes for a simple children's operetta, planning it according to the resources she could get together in the Brooklawn school community. This was new ground for her, creating a piece entirely on her own; but the place and time were right.

What she created was altogether charming, with a suggestion of boldness in the face of adversity that seemed to fit the Brooklawn setting, even allowing for the fairy tale's magic beans. "Jack and the Beanstalk" became a school project. Mothers, and some fathers, joined in to make costumes and props, including a suit for Jack's two-child cow and the flower faces for the smaller children's wayside chorus. Some of our own children enjoyed Martha's rehearsing at home and still sing, nostalgically, the principal theme, in which the chorus reinforces Jack's faltering resolve to accept the tinker/magician's offer:

> The beans are magic; his tale is true;
> Some wild adventure is promised you.
> Don't fear misfortune or mother's tears.
> The wealth that you need will be yours indeed;
> They're magic beans.

It was a unique effort for Martha, writing both words and music. Some of our children encouraged her to try to find a publisher, but she never did; and she never wrote anything else like it. Her musical talent was primarily in creating effective performance, including adaptation of what someone else had composed.

≪⌾≫

Martha's tenure at Brooklawn turned out to be only one year. The following summer, the Cherry Hill district had a place for her in elementary school music and, after two years, in the superb Music Department at Cherry Hill High School East. That department was in its heyday, with three teachers in vocal music as well as a full instrumental staff. Cherry Hill East had an enrollment of over four thousand drawn from the eastern side of the township, largely from homes where the parents were enterprising, advantaged, and mostly professional people.

Martha was quickly involved in adding choral groups. She pioneered the Belles of East, a girls' ensemble that was an instant hit when it went out spreading brightness in hospitals and convalescent homes and promoting the school in a range of settings. In matching evening dresses, each girl with a pair of English handbells, the Belles sang a selection of hit songs of the day—trenchant songs of the '60s and '70s— that they themselves arranged for accompaniment with handbells. This was Martha's idea; she provided the impetus and the Belles became self-perpetuating through successive school generations.

As Martha's years at East unfolded, the school was passing the peak of its prosperity. The district's budget began to tighten. At East, Martha's colleague who chaired the Music Department moved up to the district level and the other colleague left Cherry Hill. For vocal music, Martha now had the whole responsibility.

$\infty\infty$

My strong image comes from a winter holiday concert. We arrive as the parking lot is already filled, the building hulking dark in the December dusk against a few sunset embers in the west. Students are converging on the lighted doors to the music wing, some already in choir robes that flap as they hurry along, giving dusky glimpses of Cherry Hill East's crimson and white. Martha leaves me to hurry along too—allowing me some minutes to enjoy the crisp air, last daylight, and a bustle that I don't need to be part of. Then I lock the car and walk toward the brightly-lit main entrance.

In the foyer area outside the closed auditorium doors there is a dense cluster of people in bright winter wraps, some talking, some listening. A brass ensemble is just finishing a holiday selection. As I work my way closer, the brass players are leaving and a madrigal group in colorful Renaissance costumes is replacing them. This would be one of Martha's groups, trained to take cues from their own leader, blending their parts in the pure, straight tones of madrigal harmony. I wish that the background noise were less so that I could hear them better; but it is all part of the holiday mood.

Inside the auditorium I find a seat toward the back and exchange waves and greetings with a few of Martha's colleagues whom I know. A border with a holiday theme in greens and reds decorates the wide stage. Down front, whole sections are set aside for the various choral groups: the *varsity* men identifiable by their black suits and the girls in evening gowns.

The first part of the program is instrumental. When it's time for the vocal part, the wide curtain is left open. Bleachers are moved forward, occupying the entire stage and pressing out to the wings. As the auditorium lights dim, the freshman chorus in bright red robes is filing onstage from the left entrance. I see Martha down below. She looks small, but poised and commanding in her white bodice and flowing skirt of black lace over rose. Her hair, now entirely white, lets me follow her easily as she moves. She wouldn't think of dyeing it, and I agree. It adds beauty as well as distinction to her appearance.

She waits now without moving, while her young singers take their places. All must be motionless, all eyes on her. Then she raises her hands, nods slightly to her student accompanist at the piano, and with her first stroke, the sound reaches me like a single, blended voice. These are freshmen! How does she do it? I know, because I've been with her all the way. I know there will be no exaggerated gestures, no wide-sweeping arm movements.

"It's the eyes," she says to her singers. "Feel it and show it in your eyes!" And those eyes need to be on her, not buried in music. For these school choruses, she won't let them have music. By the time of the last rehearsal before performance, the music must all be in their heads and in their vocal cords, the harmonies felt, so that they flow out naturally. She won't ask too much of freshmen, but the varsity—the most advanced chorus—tackles difficult music and performs most of it *a capella*, without accompaniment.

The concert moves toward its finish. As each group files down off the bleachers, draining to one side, the next flows in from the other, all in orderly silence. It's only afterward that Martha tells me how one of the second sopranos passed out in the middle of a number, and the girls on each side closed up (as she'd trained them to do); while a teacher and the stage hands behind scenes helped the soprano off the bleacher. In the audience, few people had any idea that something unusual had happened.

The holiday concert finishes with a tradition that isn't in the printed program. It might seem curious, in this community surrounding and supporting Cherry Hill High School East that is strongly Jewish. The tradition is to close, with all the choruses massed on stage and joined by former students and anyone else who wishes to take part, in a rousing, reverberating rendition of the "Hallelujah Chorus" from Handel's *Messiah*. For this, Martha has all the voice power she could wish; and I, on my feet with the entire audience, feel the rush of exaltation, head to toe. What a finale; and what a send-off into the frosty, star-spangled night!

25

Who Is That Man
in the Picture?

2011

How to chart the progress of this disease? Each day, I look for signs; occasionally, a few seem to be pointing up, but most are pointing down. We continue with the coconut oil in cereal every morning. Is it helping with cognition? Is it, at least, slowing Martha's descent? With Alzheimer's, certainly at this stage, there are no precise measurements to be taken and even few telltale signs of what is happening to the brain. For Martha, we can have little doubt that the insidious "plaques" and "tangles" are there and are progressively worsening. Of the mass of marvelously, mysteriously functioning brain cells, distributed among all the critically integrated areas of the brain, billions are dying or dead. How many more each day? Is there a steady drumbeat of attrition?

For Martha and me, as for many people, there was no distinct crossing of a line. The early faltering of her brain seemed what many aging people experience. Plain kindness would block making comments to draw attention to it. And there was nothing, really, to be done. If medical science had offered us a specific diagnosis and been able to point us to a specific course of treatment, however difficult—something like chemotherapy or radiation for a cancer—that would have been different There would have been a clear threat to health, a disease to understand, to talk about and struggle against.

We understand from experts that definitive proof that a person is a victim of Alzheimer's is possible only by examining the brain after death. There are techniques of live imaging that reveal the dreaded plaques, but we read that research has found plaques in some brains apparently functioning normally to the end of life. The huge and growing threat of this disease is being met by intensive research in many centers worldwide. Our long-range hope has to be that better understanding of how and why Alzheimer's develops may bring discoveries of how to counter, or even reverse its development.

Martha and I, in our small, immediate sphere, continue with her medications. On a recent visit, our family doctor checked her over thoroughly and found everything physically functioning well. As always, he urged me to take care of myself, as well as of her.

∞∞

Among the most difficult things to cope with in this illness have been illusions or hallucinations. Our apartment at Lions Gate looks out from second-floor windows on a patch of woods dominated by a large tree, taller than the three-story building. I enjoy

watching it as it moves through the cycle of seasons—
bare branches budding, leafing, filling out in fulsome
green, then turning shades of orange-red, then brown,
letting the dry leaves go on autumn wind, to trace again
bare branches on blue sky. For Martha, it's been hard to
tell what the tree means or whether she distinguishes it
from others in view. She has sometimes seemed to see
people in the tree, maybe in the shadows under large
branches. Whoever or whatever they may be, they have
appeared to carry a vague menace. Understandably, this
has been mainly after dark. It has sometimes made
her restless, prompting her to get up and move back
and forth, staring out the windows, gesturing with a
shaking hand.

It is especially frustrating that in Martha's case, the
Alzheimer's began to impair rather early the part of
her brain associated with speech. She has shared the
frustration, as she sometimes has tried to explain what
it was that she saw, who it was who was coming, or what
was going to happen. If I ask her to repeat what she said,
hoping to catch a few more words, she would seem to
have forgotten and wouldn't try, but still would show
annoyance that I wasn't following her. The annoyance
might break out in tears, perhaps very suddenly. I may
try to calm and reassure her, while admitting that I can't
understand what she is saying. However, such efforts
at reassurance may provoke her further, bringing on
flashes of anger.

When we go down to dinner, if she is in a troubled
mood she may call out to anyone we see on the way,
whether a fellow resident, a staff person, or someone

from outside who is visiting or just making a delivery. The person she calls to may recognize the difficulty and pretend not to hear; or he or she may come over. Then Martha will say something, certain to be only partly intelligible at best. Other residents, knowing her condition, may just make some reassuring remark, to which I can appreciatively respond while we move on. Martha's redeeming feature is her generous disposition that will always return a smile when anyone speaks to her, however little she may understand of what was said.

✺

What about recognition of people? Back in Rossmoor, when we were preparing to move to Lions Gate, Martha showed an interest in doing something with a stack of family pictures that had accumulated in her desk. She found a couple of partially-filled albums, and I was glad to encourage her to mount the pictures in whatever random order she chose. Now Sylvia, on one of her visits, put an album in Martha's lap and began to turn the pages.

"Who is this person? Who is that?"

On some pages were old family photographs; I hardly knew who the people were, myself. Then, there was a picture of my cousin George. We had visited George briefly in New York City years ago, before he died. He was an artist, and from his estate I secured two abstract paintings that we hung on the wall of our living room; but no one had been speaking recently about him.

Martha looked at the photo in the album. "George," she said and, twisting around, pointed up at his paintings. Who would have thought her memory could bring up that recollection and make that association?

On the other hand—and this was on another day—there was a picture of me in the album. When Sylvia asked, "Who is that man in the picture?" Martha said, "My husband, Donald." She never called me Donald, and seemed to be making no connection with the person who was watching from three or four feet away.

Then it was Sylvia's turn in the recognition game. Martha appeared unable to recognize any of her children that day until, in one photograph, she identified Donna. A page or two later, there was a large studio photo of Sylvia herself as a one-year-old. "That's Sylvia," Martha said. She remembered the baby but, again, made no identification with the affectionate adult daughter who was turning the pages beside her.

26

Mrs. Fletcher, Please, Can You Come?

1988, 1996

Martha and I retired from teaching in 1986, but she kept on privately with a few voice students who particularly interested her. There was Julie (not her real name), who had a beautiful voice, but also emotional problems. Julie feuded with her mother; her father was not in the picture. She was trying to get more education or a job and was living here and there.

One night, we had a call; it was a counselor of some sort in Philadelphia. Julie had attempted suicide, had been hysterical. Somewhat calmer now, she wanted to talk to Martha. The counselor put her on the phone.

"Mrs. Fletcher, please. Can you come? I need you. I need to talk to you and to Mr. Fletcher too. Can you come, both of you?"

We could and did, late as it was. We found Julie calm, subdued. She held Martha in a long embrace; there were tears, and we talked long and quietly. She wanted to cling and to be told that she was right; but Martha took the mother's part. Julie must be strong. She was the one who had broken with her mother; she must be the one to reconcile. No, she wasn't alone and abandoned. We would be there; but it was her mother that she needed, and who needed her.

When at last we were on our way home, there wasn't much wish to talk more. I had added to Julie a pastoral part, knowing the foundation of faith that she had and wanting to help her face the finality of suicide.

After a long silence while we reached and crossed the bridge back to New Jersey, Martha spoke, wondering if Julie had really wanted to end her life. I doubted it, but I was glad that she had turned to Martha—to both of us, as Martha corrected me. I said that, anyway, I thought Martha had convinced her to get back to her mother.

Julie did get back. There were other stormy times; but she began to find herself, to make her way, and to have some peace. In time, her mother divorced, and after that, both she and Julie found steady male companionship that suited their very different personalities.

⁓⁓⁓

We moved an hour north to Rossmoor, an over-55 community. I became pastor of the community church and Martha, organist and music director. We hadn't been teamed up like that since our time in Antofagasta, Chile, almost forty years earlier. In Rossmoor, our congregation shared the use of the meeting house with other faith groups and many public gatherings. The versatile building had been designed along the lines of a New England meeting house or congregational church, with a white spire above its single main door, tall, clear-glass windows, and a classic, plain interior.

Martha and I sparked a campaign to replace the aging electric organ with the many voices of a Hammond 36, its powerful speakers mounted in openings on each side of the proscenium.

On the organ bench, Martha's musical self had full range. I knew that in services, the fabric of worship would be woven together, her improvised transitions moving us seamlessly from one part to the next. And the remarkable capabilities of the Hammond, all in reach of Martha's hands and feet, could speak in awesome power or slender, delicate tone. There was even a choral stop that sounded like human voices wonderfully blended.

I can't say that the scene I'm going to describe is literal fact, happening on a specific day, but it is woven from my memories of how it was. I can envision us going together to the meeting house, as we often did— Martha wanting to practice, and I always with work to do in my office that was on the second floor, adjoining the rear balcony of the auditorium.

When I think she is probably finished, I go to look from the balcony. She is putting her music away in the organ bench. A shaft of the westering sun coming through the high window opposite is catching her white hair, making it almost glow.

"Wait," I call. "Just one thing before we go. Let me hear 'God of Our Life, Through All the Circling Years.'"

It is a great hymn, written by Hugh Thompson Kerr in 1916, under the lowering of World War I. My dad discovered it, and it became a favorite of our family, and from there, a sort of signature hymn of Martha's and my family later on. Martha gets back on the bench.

She chooses a serene combination of stops, and the first chords well up in the autumn light that is filling the empty auditorium.

> God of our life, through all the circling years,
> We trust in Thee;
> In all the past, through all our hopes and fears,
> Thy hand we see.

Martha's foot moves on the swell pedal. The tone grows richer and deeper, then begins to subside.

> With each new day, when morning lifts the veil,
> We own Thy mercies, Lord, which never fail.

"Beautiful!" I call down. "Now the last stanza; give it everything!" Of course no one is singing, but the words speak eloquently in my mind. These days, we don't use the archaic "Thou" and "Thee", but I question if anyone out there is writing hymns as purely lyrical as Kerr's text. Down at the console, Martha's quick hands are selecting combinations and stops. Then the wonderful sound comes, filling powerfully every crevice of the high-ceilinged hall.

> God of the coming years, through paths unknown
> We follow Thee;
> When we are strong, Lord, leave us not alone;
> Our refuge be.

"When we are strong..." The music seems to be shaking the balcony; I know that I am shaking, as those words always shake me.

Be Thou for us in life our daily bread,
Our heart's true home when all our years have
    sped.

The magnificent sound ends; the organ goes silent. Orange and red-gold light, refracted off Rossmoor's glorious autumn foliage outside the western windows, floods the room. I am aware of pain in my fingers where they grip the balcony rail and of wetness on my cheeks.

Be Thou for us in life our daily bread,
Our heart's true home when all our years have
    sped.

Martha had to be feeling the same emotion, the way she played that hymn. When I meet her downstairs in the foyer, I can see that her eyes, too, are wet.

27

My Wife Asks Me, "Who Are You?"

2011

The working and not-working of Martha's brain and its impact on her personality at this stage show up distinctly in some of my notes.

Thursday, April 14, 2011
Alan and Ron were visiting; when I came back at 1:00 p.m. they were there. Martha greeted me, broke down in tears, and clung to me. We had lunch in Lions Gate's Bistro. Martha, still sad and tearful, beckoned to everyone she saw, telling one person that she was going to die.

In the evening, as just she and I were returning from dinner, she was obsessed with an idea of needing to go outside. We walked as we were—without coats—some distance in the parking lot. At bedtime, she wouldn't go to bed—finally, partly undressed, sitting on the edge of the bed, she was determined to put her shoes on again. "You can't wear your shoes to bed." "I always go to bed with my shoes on," she retorted.

I put the shoes far under a rocking chair, then went to the walk-in closet, turning my back to see what she would do. When I looked again, she was in bed; turned away from me. I kissed her on the temple. Returning an hour later, I found the shoes on top of the covers at the foot of the bed. She had slipped out, gotten them, and put them there; then she slipped in again and was sound asleep. She had made her statement.

Thursday, April 21

Martha was cheerful and at ease in the afternoon, but her mood darkened later. I got her to walk (always with the walker) to dinner with some difficulty, then sat at a table for two. After we were home, she was restless, didn't want the TV, and began having her ideas that someone was outside. We walked our corridor, up and down all the way, three times. About 8:30 p.m., I put the wheelchair, brakes set, against our door (no way to lock the door against opening from inside). She refused to get ready for bed. After 10:00, I said I was going to turn in; she watched me, still refusing, insisting on something about someone coming. I left her sitting on the sofa in the living room. She was still there at 11:00. I set my alarm for 12:00; she was still there. She would come to the bedroom from time to time, as I was fitfully aware, and I kept checking on her off and on. At 4:20 a.m., she finally came to bed and let me cover her up—quite peaceful and affectionate. The obsession with *people* who were coming, and her need to go somewhere had at last subsided (when it drives her, it can give amazing stamina and strength).

Tuesday, May 3

Martha was unusually positive and serene; she walked to the elevator and first-floor corridor to our mailbox—only a moment tearful but very shaky later, so we used the wheelchair to go to dinner. Coming back, she was asking about home but seemed satisfied with my explanations about this home. She sat down on the sofa, then looked up at me and asked, "Just who are you?" I sat beside her and said, "Do you know who Don is? I'm Don."

With a bit more of this, she raised no more questions. I went on speaking about former homes, relating them to the births of our children, one by one. Each time, Martha nodded quite firmly, seeming to remember. So I spoke about the book I was working on and—for the first time—very plainly about her illness, using the Alzheimer's name. She didn't nod, but I think she had some idea. All through this talk she was affectionate, wanting to kiss after each part; then went to bed serenely about 8:30 p.m.

Wednesday, July 13

As the dinner hour approached, Martha was very resistant. I let some time pass, then was able to get her on her feet and started out with the walker. Going up the sloping passageway from our building she asked, "Who are you?" I made a simple answer. At dinner, sitting with

two friends, she asked me the same question—
fortunately not very loud, and the friends didn't
hear well. Returning after dinner, she wanted to
know where we were going. I explained about
our apartment home. Later, sitting on the sofa,
she seemed in doubt about who we are. I was
telling her about herself: Martha Bradway, then
M. B. Fletcher; then began to speak about the
children—asked her the name of the oldest—
silence. I began to go through the list, one by
one. She said she didn't understand, acted as if
she were hearing the names of her children for
the first time. I returned to reassuring her about
us, who we are and what we are to each other.
About 9:00 p.m., she went cooperatively to bed.
Later, when I was at the computer in the den,
she appeared in the doorway. When I got her
back in bed and followed soon after, she was
very affectionate, saying, "I love you."

Two evenings later, I was speaking to
Martha about our children, and again, she
wasn't responding to their names; but as we got
up from the sofa to go to the bedroom, she went
over to touch a pair of their bronzed baby shoes
on a lamp table, making some speech sound
that seemed to show she associated these with
what I had been saying.

Tuesday, August 23

The day began well; Martha was up, and
had her breakfast with our aide before I left
at 9:50 a.m. for my Tuesday morning support
group. When I was back at 1:00 p.m., she ate a
good lunch, still in a positive frame of mind and

was loving toward me. With some misgiving, I had made an appointment for 2:00 p.m. to have her hair washed and cut at our salon in Lions Gate. It worked out well. Martha agreed to go, walked the series of long corridors to the salon and even submitted—with minimal protest—to being tipped far back, her head at the edge of a sink for the shampoo. I stayed standing close by, then walked her home.

Her positive, affectionate mood held up through a nap and dinner preparation, putting up only a small resistance to getting on her feet, taking the walker, and starting off again down the corridor. We were meeting a couple of friends for dinner, something I don't often risk trying, but it proved pleasant—just a little anxiety to be sure I would stay with her, as we went home.

In the evening, after I turned off the TV—news packed with Tripoli falling to the opposition, hurricane Irene advancing toward the East Coast, and a 5.8 earthquake in Virginia (that we didn't feel, as we were walking to the hair appointment)—Martha was very loving and unusually clear. She continued responsive as I talked about having each other and about the children and grandchildren, then went easily to the bedroom and so to bed. What a good day!

☙❧

Back on May 19, sitting in the big chair at Marilyn and Dale's home, I was reflecting on what was happening to us two, wanting to mark the day, our 69th wedding anniversary. The result was a lyric poem.

Anniversary

This much is left, my love. I will not ask
For more; just let me have it, still, this way:
Your smile, even your tears, when I have been
Away and you come reaching out to me.
Love, it's still you—it is—the darker times,
Flashes of anger where the shadow looms,
Creeping across your brightness, these are not,
Not you, more than the ominous shapes
That move outside our twilight windows. Love,
Let me feel your breathing warmth, your lifted
      lips
Turning to mine. See, we are here, we two,
Sixty-nine years. Let it be so. I know
It will not be. The eclipsing shadow will
Not stop before darkness; but I'll raise this
      stone,
This marker to remember: sixty-nine.

28

Easing Martha through Her Days and Nights

2012

We seem to be entering on a further phase of Martha's illness. A positive aspect is that the illusions have largely disappeared. She still looks out the windows, and will go over to them when she can, but seldom seems to have seen anything disturbing out there. When I comment to her on the traffic and on the changing daylight as afternoon draws toward evening, she may respond, or seem to, but without alarm. There is rarely an idea of people coming—some vaguely sinister *they* whom she expects. Nor are we needing to go somewhere urgently, as before.

We still quite often have a *sundown* change of mood in late afternoon; but it is likely to show itself simply as resistance—sometimes categorical resistance—to getting ready and to going down to dinner. Our evening aide—who comes at 5:00—may run into that resistance, testing her and my combined ingenuity to find a way around it. Occasionally, we are completely baffled. It's good that, being where we are, I can call down to the desk and have a dinner sent up for Martha (the aide helps her with that), while I go to the dining room alone. That is a solution, but one that feels like defeat. The daily dinner hour is the prime social event in a community like Lions Gate, and Martha usually enters into it once she is there, smiling and waving to people she knows, or thinks she knows.

The other day, we were on our way down, our aide pushing the wheelchair and I walking beside it, after some resistance from Martha. I was keeping up a monologue meant to be reassuring. "So here we are," I said. "Going to dinner, the three of us..." Quickly and with unusual clarity, Martha responded, "Who's going to cook?" Once in a while, startlingly, those impulses in the brain get through.

There is another emerging problem that affects our dinner hour. Martha's control of her hands is becoming so erratic that eating on her own can be almost impossible. This is not a consistent trembling or shaking, but convulsive, unpredictable movement. And it varies, being some days worse than others.

In the dining room, I prefer to have a table for two, although friends are understanding and insist that they don't mind at all if Martha's efforts with her implements are awkward or even if she simply takes up a difficult mouthful with her fingers. At issue is a dining room rule that I myself endorsed, sitting on our nine-member residents' council. Concerned about the atmosphere of our dining rooms—particularly as perceived by visiting, prospective residents—we agreed that no resident requiring to be fed by another person should eat in the dining rooms. For that condition, one must take the meal in his or her apartment or move to the assisted living or the skilled nursing facility. This is what I will be facing with Martha, when she is no longer able to control that fork or spoon at all. I already do the knife work, cutting up meat and anything else on her plate that needs bite-size reduction.

About mobility, I've described the drastic effect of Martha's fall and hip fracture, how the trauma left her, at first, confined to a wheelchair; then, how we gradually got her walking again. She was even able to do the long corridors from our apartment to the dining rooms on foot, with the help of a simple walker. Now that regained ground has largely been lost.

Around the apartment on good days, she may get to her feet with only a little help and walk short distances quite firmly with just the support of someone holding her arm; although even on such days, we use the walker for going from room to room. In the corridors, or to and from the car, it must always be the wheelchair. Even in the apartment, on days when Martha is shakier and we help her to her feet, her legs—particularly the left leg (not the one with the replaced hip), for whatever reason—can show an alarming tendency to buckle, so that extreme care must be taken for emergency support. How proud we humans are of our ability to walk on our hind legs, and what a precarious skill that is!

Currently, Martha's day is not very long. In the morning, she tends to sleep in or, even if awake and just dozing intermittently, to resist any proposal to get up. The aide comes seven days a week, from 9:00 a.m. to 1:00 p.m., and only rarely finds Martha up and perhaps sitting at the breakfast table in her robe. What is more usual is that the clock moves on to 11:00 or 11:30 in the morning and nothing the aide can think of persuades Martha to loosen her determined grip on the covers and to swing her legs out peacefully to leave the bed. When I come home at 1:00, I may be told that she finished breakfast only a half hour before.

When the aide leaves, I go about preparing a simple lunch, perhaps primarily for me, although Martha always shares it, surprising me sometimes by how heartily she eats. After lunch and a brief kitchen clean-up, I help her move to her favorite place at the end of the sofa that is nearer the windows, settling in next to her for what is usually a quite long afternoon nap. My concern on most days is that Martha tends to keep on dozing after nap time, as the afternoon wears away. I have tried with little success to find activities that might catch and hold her attention, anything to look at or for me to talk about.

With the approach of 5:00 p.m., whatever way we have passed the time, I try to prepare for the arrival of our evening aide and the routine of getting ready and going down to dinner. I've mentioned the *sundown* phenomenon and the resistance that we are likely to encounter. If that can be successfully dealt with, we are on our way, threading the corridors to the dining room. After dinner we return to our apartment. Lately our pattern, after watching TV news for a half hour or so, has been for the aide to take Martha back to the common rooms, enjoying some distraction and contact with people. They return around 8:30, and I reassure

Martha that I am there. That seems to be enough for her to go willingly on her way to the bedroom.

By 9:00 p.m., when the aide leaves, Martha is tucked in bed. Since she sleeps well, we are still able to share our bed, that is a comfort to me and I think to her also. So, now I take over, assuring her that it is just the two of us together, as we've always been. I am close by, in the next room. She can call and I'll hear her; but I don't want her to try to get up without me. For my assurance, the string of the bed alarm is clipped to the shoulder of her nightgown. If she does start to get up, that string will pull a magnet away from the alarm, where it hangs on the bed's headboard, and the insistent beeping will alert me anywhere in the apartment—or during the night, although I'm a sound sleeper, it will waken me.

Nighttime is to be treasured after Martha's short day—especially that moment when I slide in at my side of the bed. She realizes I am there, and stirs, whether she actually wakes up or not. For me, what matters is the warmth and closeness, feeling her breathing, touching her face. I can tell myself it won't last—that the change looms, when I can't have her with me like this any longer—when she'll require a different kind of care. I can't hold back the eclipsing shadow—I know that. But in our bedroom, with the distant whiteness of those street lights that she likes to watch and the soft night-light beyond the bathroom door, here I can hold her now. Amen—let it be so.

29

Pain and a Need for Support

Alzheimer's is a terminal disease without pain. As I have commented, Martha and I didn't talk about it at an early stage, and later, she would seem to have been quite unaware of what was happening to her. As with others coping with the illness, it is I, as caregiver, who feel the pain and need support. Where do I turn for that?

I am not gregarious. I enjoy friendly company, and conversation that gets beyond an exchange of commonplace remarks, and I certainly am influenced by other people's ideas; but I don't naturally turn to others for emotional support. While I don't think of myself as a loner, I don't mind being alone. When I wish—or feel a need—to work something out, I look for quiet, even solitude, and if that can be in a beautiful or serene setting, so much the better.

As a minister, I am professionally religious, and I naturally feel at home in a Presbyterian (USA) context that is my heritage and training. But for spiritual support, I don't turn to ritual, creed, or cultic observance. I find my help, primarily, in reflection that may lead to moments of insight or inspiration.

My faith affirms the reality of God, who is Spirit, and of my communion, as spirit, with God. God is *transcendent*, beyond or outside of this cosmos of space and time. We only know what is within the limits of space and time—what we can observe, measure, and experience in our universe—even while we are constantly inventing instruments that extend our range of observation. These enable us to see enormous distances in outer space and minute details of inner space that are much beyond the unaided human eye. They also enable us to project our observation billions of years into the past of the universe, as well as theoretically into its future. But all such observation—all of science—is limited by and to time and space.

What has been exciting and transforming for me, in terms of faith, is precisely the advance of science, opening up to human perception the two vastnesses of space and time. I think of God as the Creator, God who transcends our space/time universe, but who brings it into being. I see in it how God's creating purpose moves with a scope I can hardly conceive. Our spiritual forebears—prophetic minds and spirits of Judaism, Christianity, and Islam, as also of the world's other great philosophic and religious traditions—lived in a much smaller world. For them, space was quite limited. The heavens were presided over by the sun and moon and a host of stars, those that their eyes could see on a clear, dark night—and all these were in a vault above the earth, or moved around the earth in stately procession. And as for time, they believed they could count back a few dozen generations, at most, to an original pair and the origin of humanity. Each tradition had its creation story—the most familiar to us being the Genesis story of the making of "the heavens and the earth" and all life in six days.

In more recent ages, religious leaders have modified and interpreted the creation stories. Yet, for me, it is modern science that has suddenly and hugely expanded our perception of the universe, and in so doing, has impressed on those of us who have such faith a radical expansion of our idea of God. It now appears to us that God, in the evolutionary process, creates life in a deliberate and seemingly circuitous way that we struggle to comprehend. Even at our present stage of human life, those few dozen generations traced back to our origin by the ancients are now seen to number in the tens of thousands. Nor is there any set beginning of humanity to be found, as the small degrees of evolution stretch into the remote past. Somewhere along the line, somehow, human consciousness—soul, spirit— has come into being. My faith affirms that all this is of God. The Transcendent, the Creator wills it to be.

Further, I must try to comprehend what my faith finds even more difficult. The process of mutation and of survival of the fittest that results in an evolution of life forms, as willed by the Creator, involves conflict, suffering, and death. As those forms evolve, they survive and continue to survive, many of them, by predation— by hunting, killing, and consuming other forms of life. This has to be part of the Creator's design, unless one declares that there is no Creator, only blind chance.

Our forebears, authors of the Bible and the scriptures of other faiths, did not have to cope with the vastness and complexity of space and time that is now part of any well-taught schoolchild's universe. Nor did they have to cope with suffering and death as being part of the Creator's purpose from the beginning. They could see death as a consequence of human sin, as in the Christian New Testament.

In pondering my faith in God, I feel, on one hand, an awesome sense of God's transcendence. The awareness of the vast scale of the universe, and of the long history and the complexity of life on this small planet Earth, makes me confess that I can't at all think like God. As the Hebrew Prophet of the Exile expressed it,

> For my thoughts are not your thoughts,
> nor are your ways my ways, says the LORD.
> For as the heavens are higher than the earth,
> so are my ways higher than your ways
> and my thoughts than your thoughts.
>
> Isaiah 55:8–9 (NRSV)

On the other hand, I believe deeply in that central insight of the Abrahamic faiths, that God loves and cares about God's creation: "You shall love the Lord your God" (Judaism); for "God is love" (Christianity); and, "Allah, most benevolent, ever merciful" (Islam). Being of God, this is transcendent love—love, total and absolute. And love, even in our faltering experience of it, must be reaching out, longing to communicate with the one who is loved. I perceive the Spirit reaching, touching, inspiring prophets, poets, and sages of our whole known range of cultures and religious traditions, wherever there is an insight that is noble and uplifting. Why has the inspiration been so fragmentary and so easily debased? This is to ask, why does our human spirit present such a mixture of good and evil, of beauty and corruption? Because God makes us free—free to choose which way to be.

I hold by faith that God, Spirit, reaches me, who am spirit—that God's wisdom and God's love are always near for me—as for this loved person whom I cherish. God loves her far better than I can, and in the ending of our pilgrimage through time, what waits for us beyond our knowing or imagining is of love—of God.

These thoughts provide, for me, both a sense of transcendence—God, utterly beyond my comprehension in wisdom, power, and compassion—and a sense of gracious nearness, almost intimacy. In these lines, written in the fall of 2011, I try to express that nearness:

Grace

Here now, this moment, You are inviting me
to experience love, absolute, quintessential,
in her whom you give
and draw away from me, to stretch thin the
  thread
that you make unbreakable.
That is love—your astounding, agonizing grace.
I thank you for it; in the tears of my wrung-dry
  heart
I thank you that this way—and only this—
I can know Love, have some inkling of
your love, that is You, grace-sprinkled on my
  pain.

30

Eternal Sea

Many years ago, May 19, 1981, I wanted to write a lyric for Martha on our anniversary, but nothing would come. I began some lines with that regret, "I have no song tonight," that became a refrain for the first two stanzas. It's the third stanza that I include here:

> Well, we will go together down the beach,
> As we have gone, holding each other's hands
> Perhaps a little tighter, as the sands
> Get softer underfoot, and the tide's reach
> Comes closer. There, at least, I know the long
> Surge and resurge of timeless waves will teach
> My love a song.

That image that welled up in mind years ago fits our life as it is now—going down the beach, this last beach by the eternal sea. I had pictured us, poetically, approaching hand in hand quite consciously that final transition. We are approaching it, and still hand in hand, as I thank God, but Martha is much deeper in than I. I can't tell anymore what awareness she may have; but my reassurance is that she still reaches out to me. Most of the time, she knows me and responds with affection—even a tearful, clinging, almost desperate affection. I pray to God that her love for me may be the last rim of brightness I can see before Alzheimer's eclipse is complete.

Does that eclipse mean surrender? No. This thing is physical. The living cells of the brain are being blocked and dying off, the lights put out successively. But the spirit—the intangible, the incorruptible person—lives.

This I believe. There is no proof. Proof belongs to the space/time cosmos, and spirit does not, as God does not. The eternal sea, in the image of the poem, is outside space and time. It transcends space/time, not restricted by the limits of this limited cosmos that we know.

That may be a bit frightening. Since early times, people have tried to find reassurance by imagining an afterlife that is like their present life, just extended in ideal terms—a paradise, a lush desert oasis, an unending banquet. This we know nothing of. We can imagine shores of whatever kind beyond the eternal sea.

What is enough is that our love goes with us—my love and Martha's, as she still responds to me—and that love, true and perfect love, awaits us beyond. Faith affirms that such is God, Author of our being, Giver of life and love. There is no obscuring, eclipsing shadow on that brightness.

Photographs

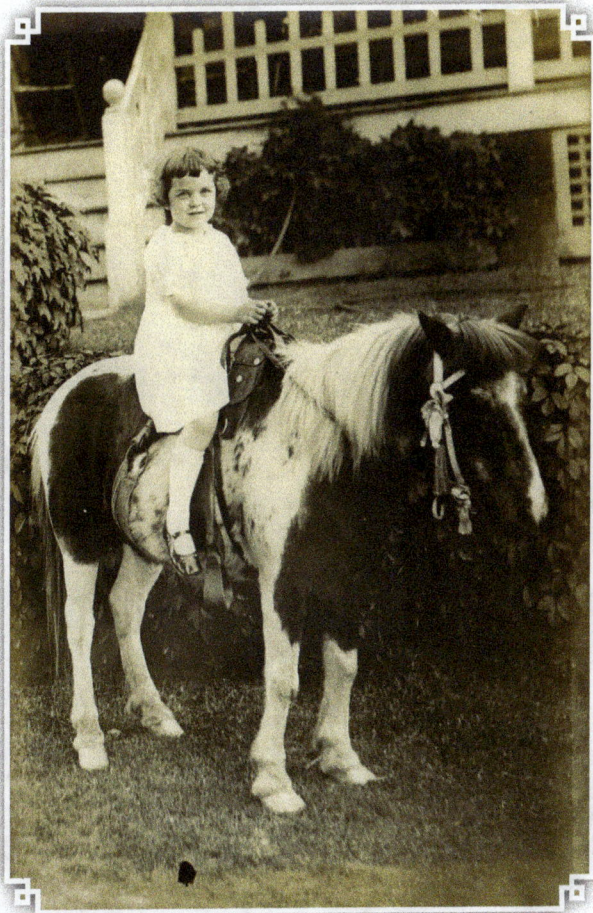

Martha at age five, 1927

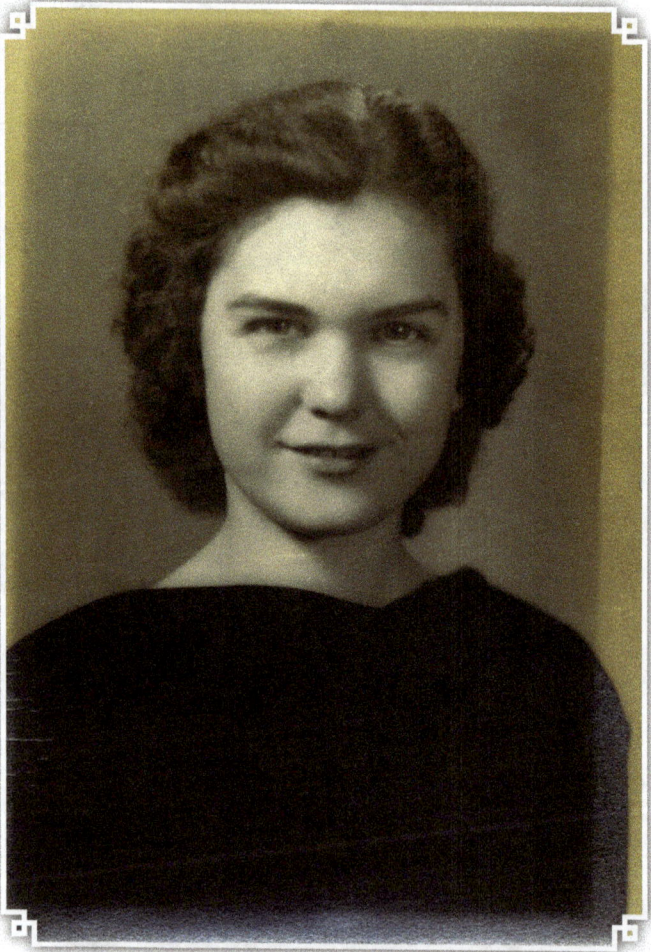

Martha as a high school senior, 1939

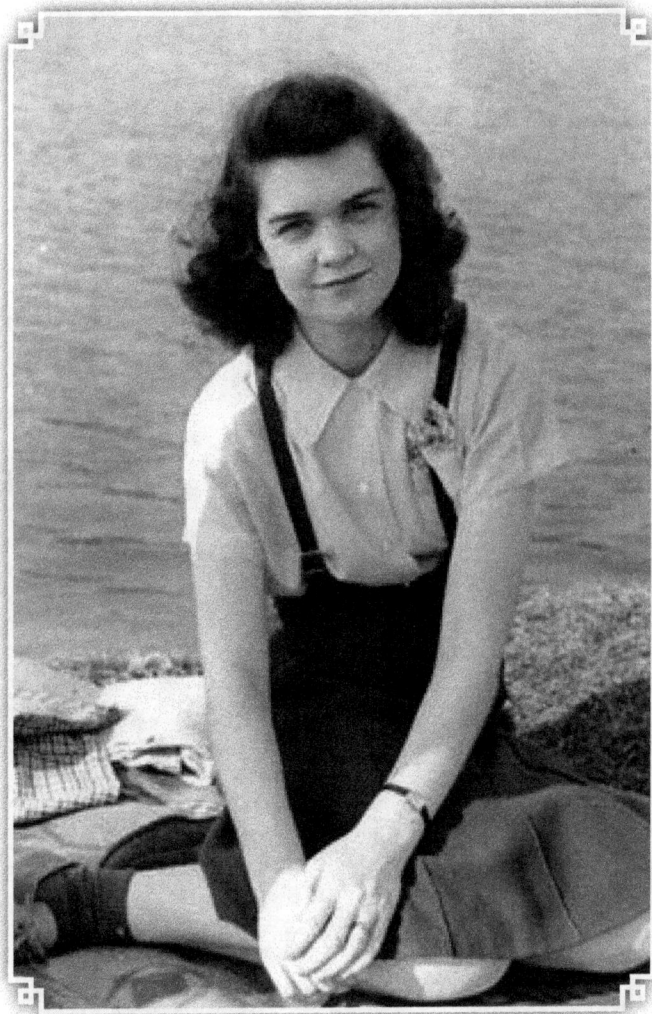

Spring of 1941; notice the Princeton ring

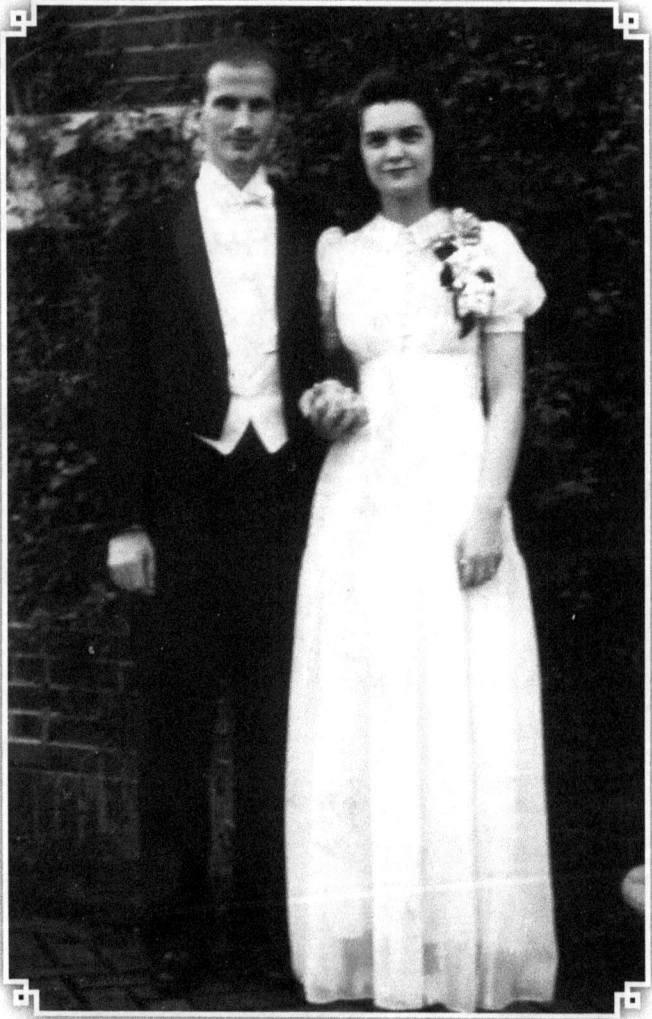

Martha and Don, dressed for a formal concert
at Westminster Choir College, 1943

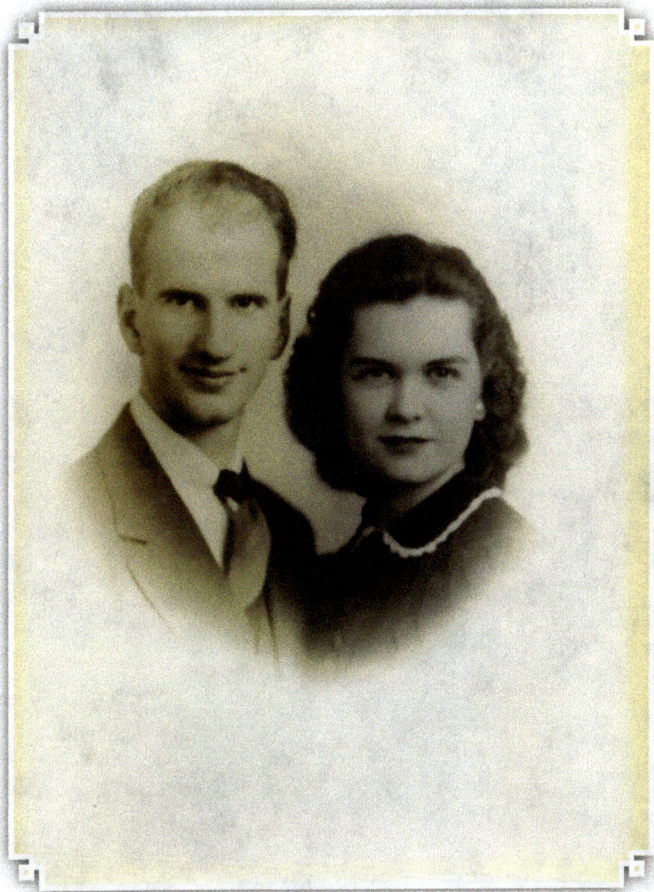

Studio photo as new missionaries, 1945

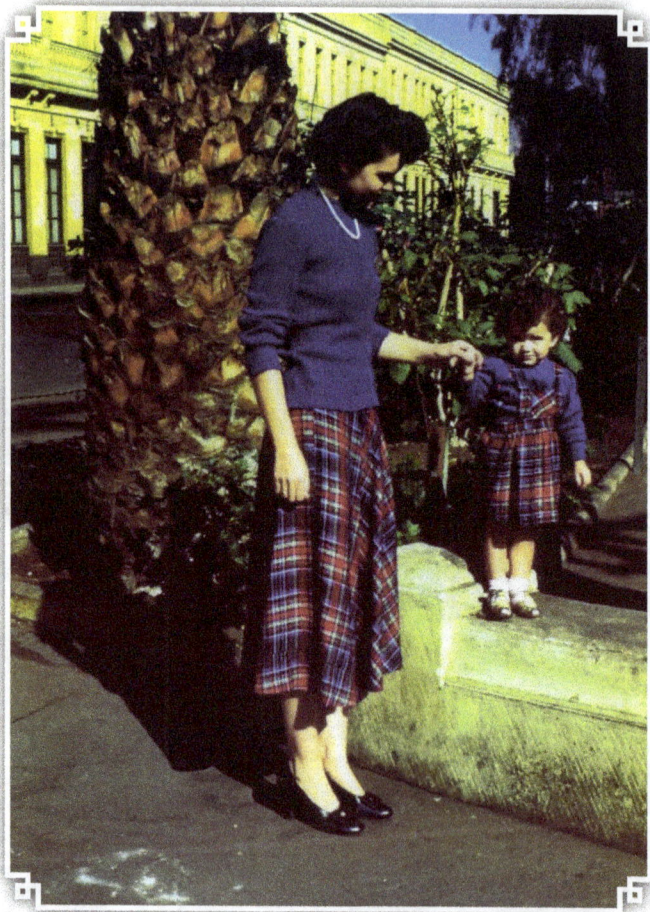

With Donna, on an avenue in Antofagasta, Chile, 1949

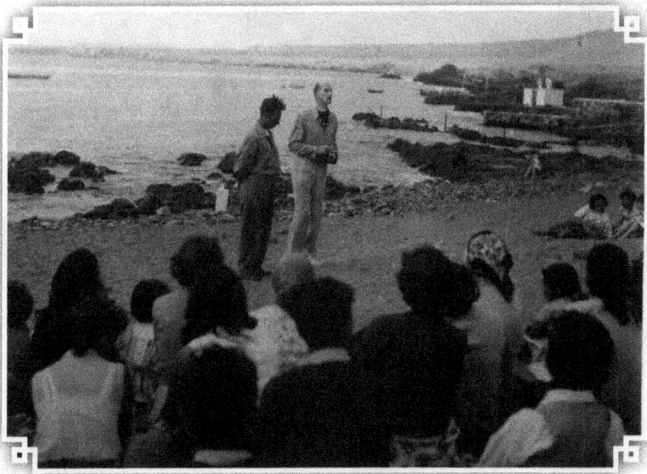

Don leading a youth group on the Antofagasta shore, 1950

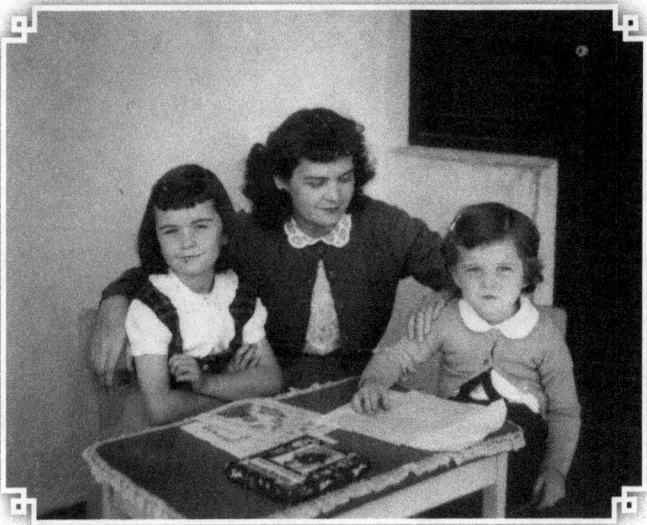

Homeschooling Donna and Sylvia, 1953

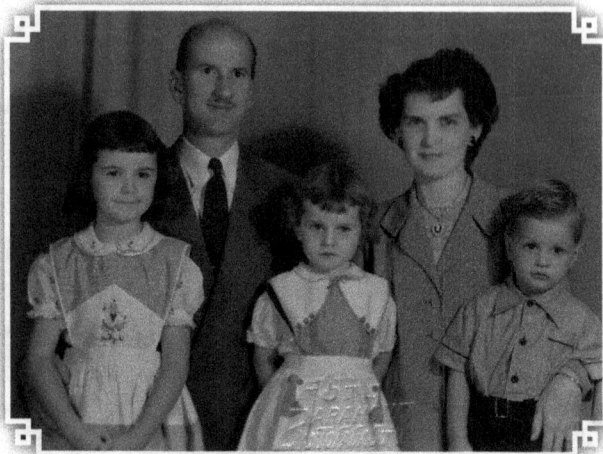

Our family of three children, 1953

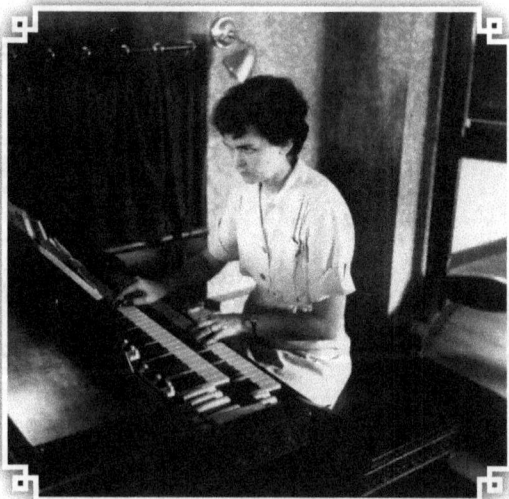

At the Hammond console in the new
Antofagasta church building, 1955

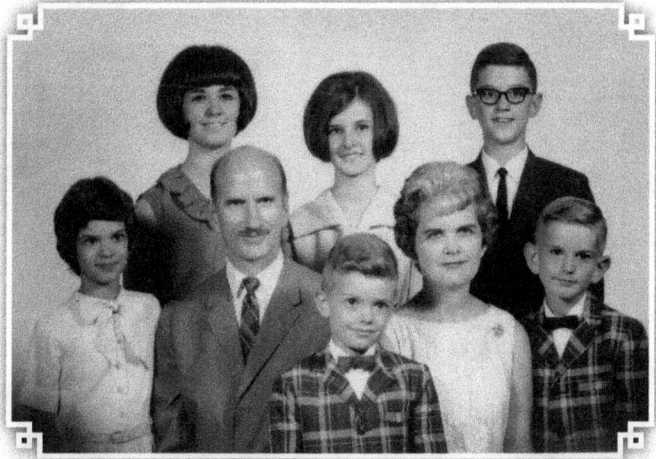

Our complete family after the move to Austin, Texas, 1960

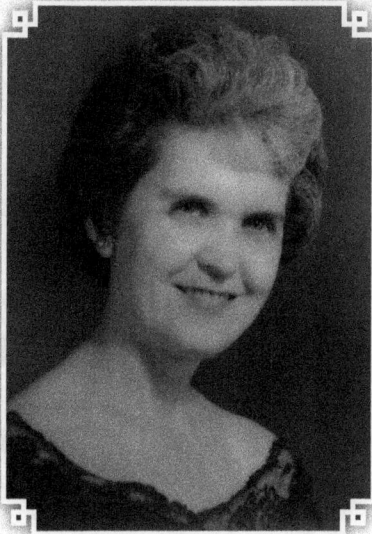

Martha at age 42; publicity photo in Austin, 1964

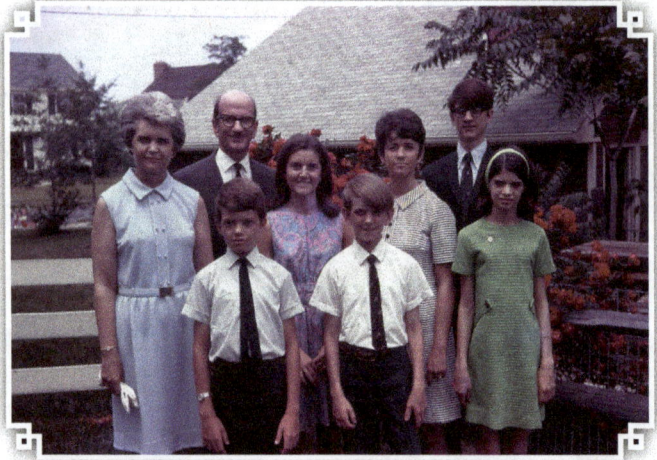

The family, at our new home in Cherry Hill, NJ, 1967

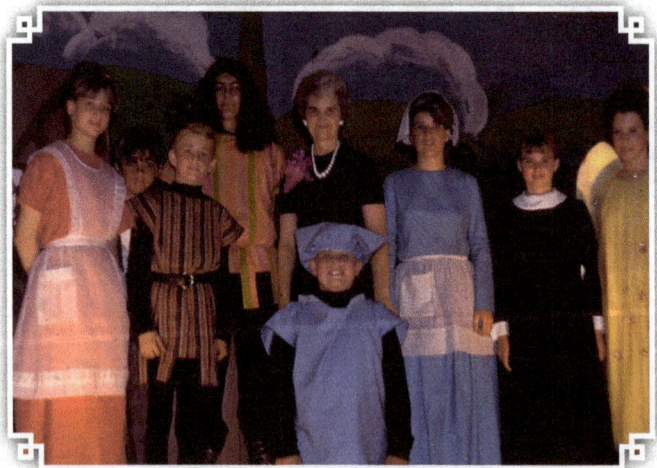

With part of the "Jack and the Beanstalk" cast, 1974

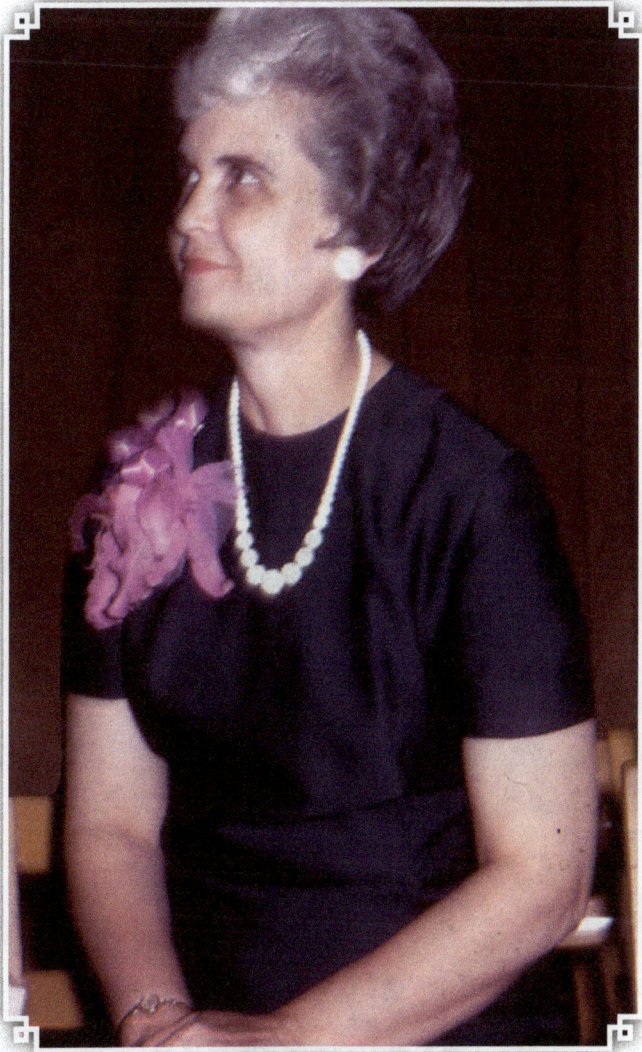

At the performance of "Jack and the
Beanstalk", Brooklawn, NJ, 1974

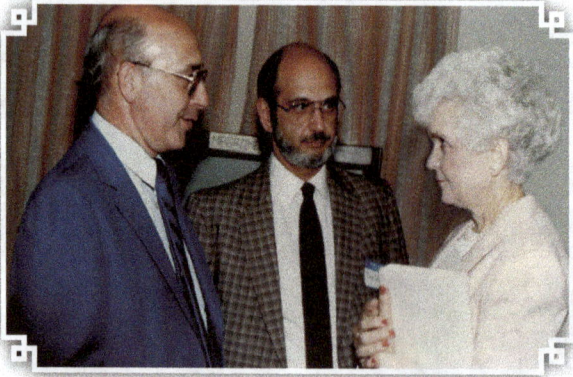

At Cherry Hill High School East, speaking
with school principals, 1984

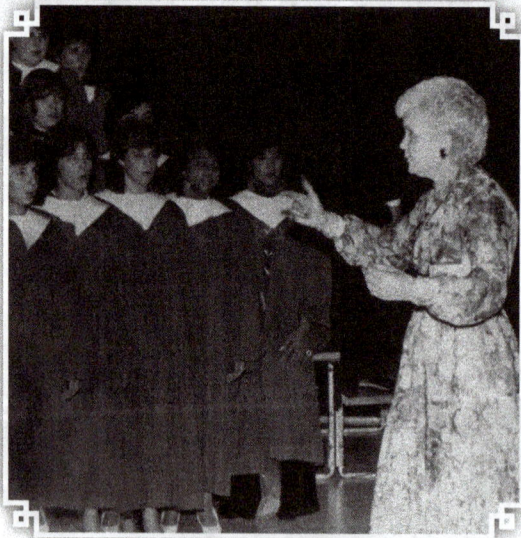

Rehearsing a choral group before concert
at Cherry Hill East, 1985

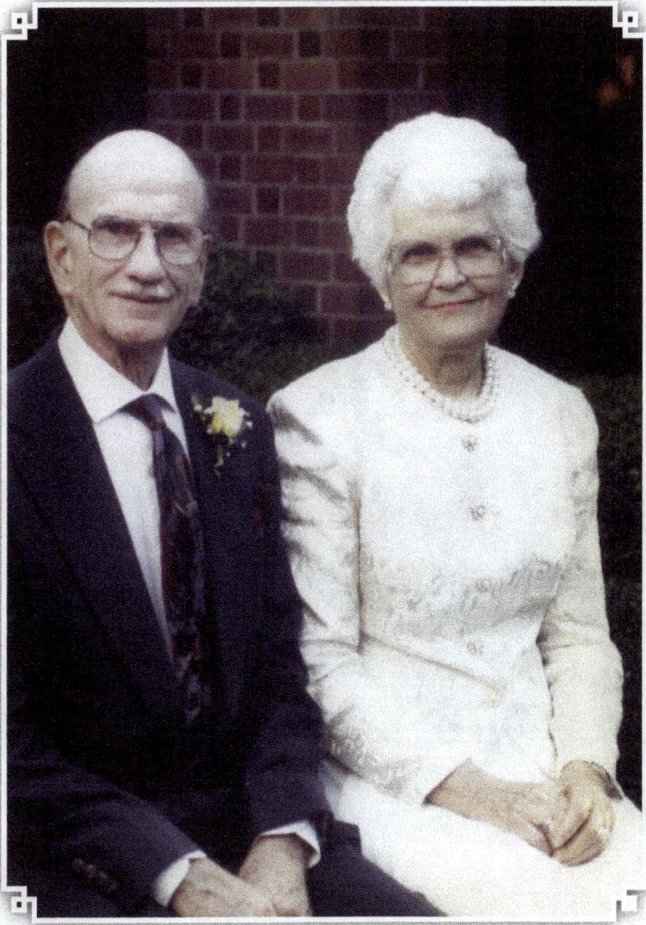

At our 50th Wedding Anniversary celebration, 1992

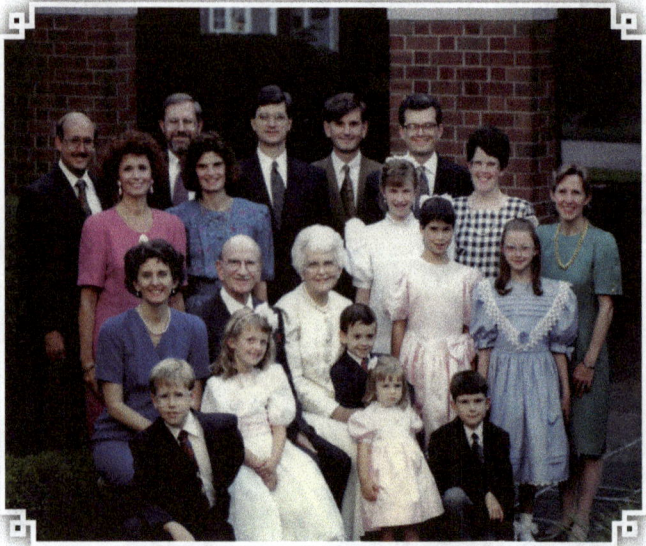

The whole family, at our 50th Anniversary, 1992

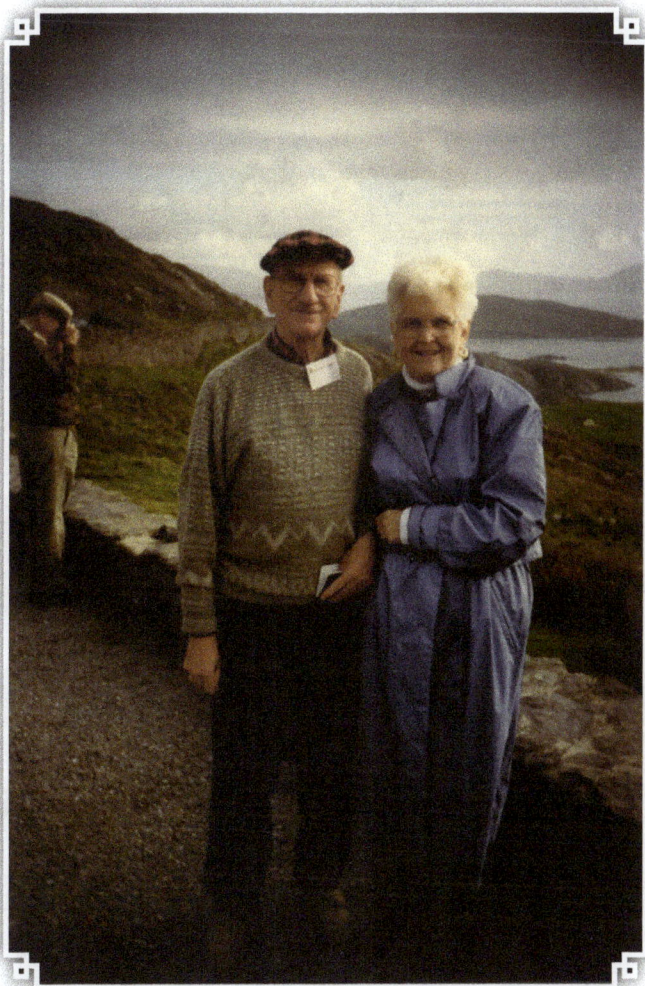

On a trip to Ireland in the later 1990's

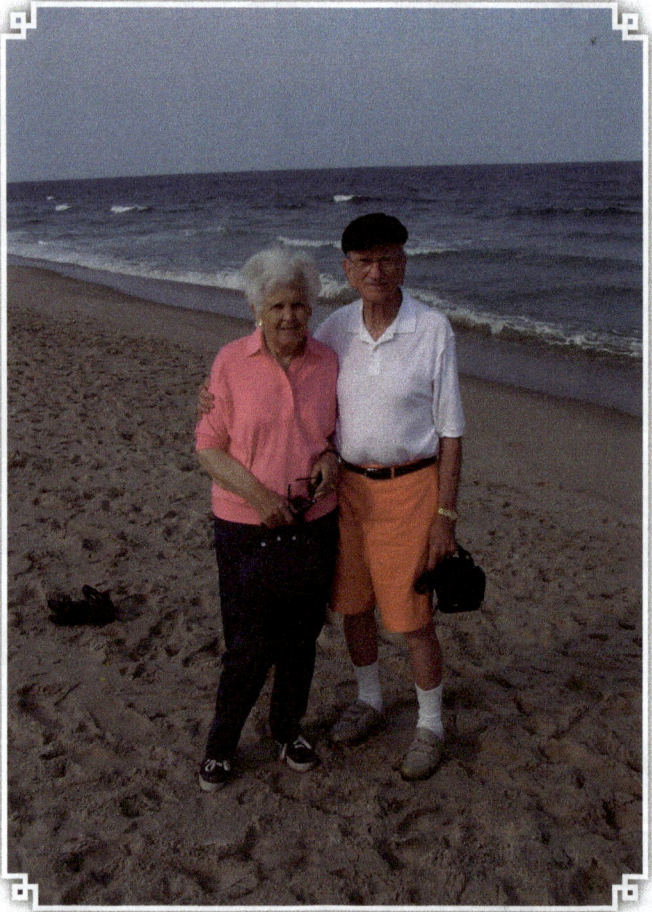

On Nantuckett Island, 2005

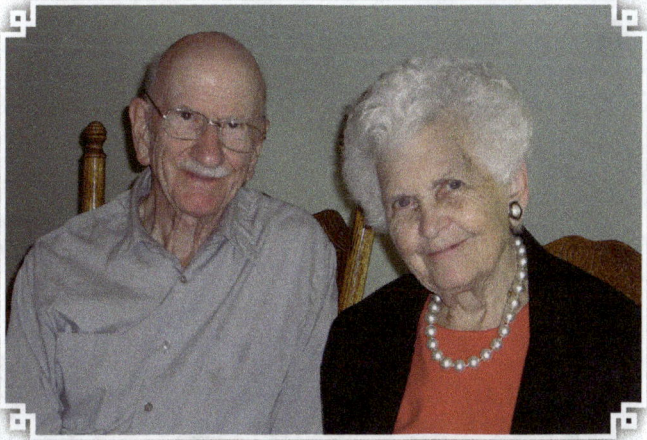

Martha and Don, 2006

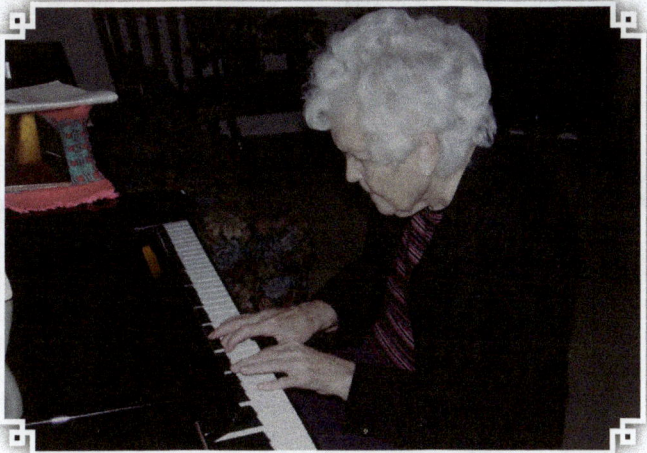

Martha, unable to play, still conveys a deep
familiarity with her keyboard, 2011

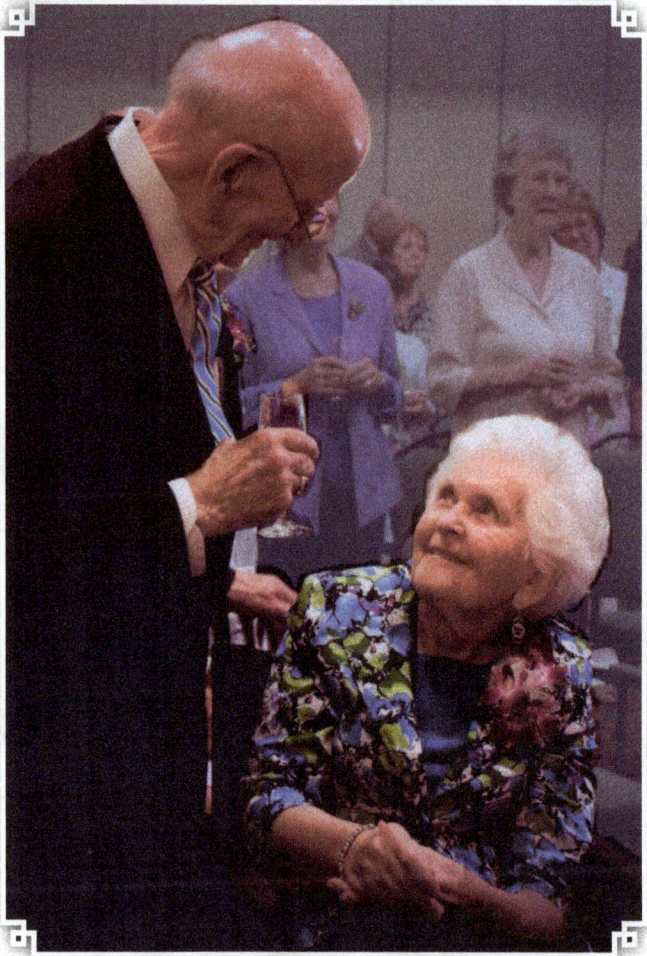

At our 70th Wedding Anniversary and
Martha's 90th Birthday, June 2012

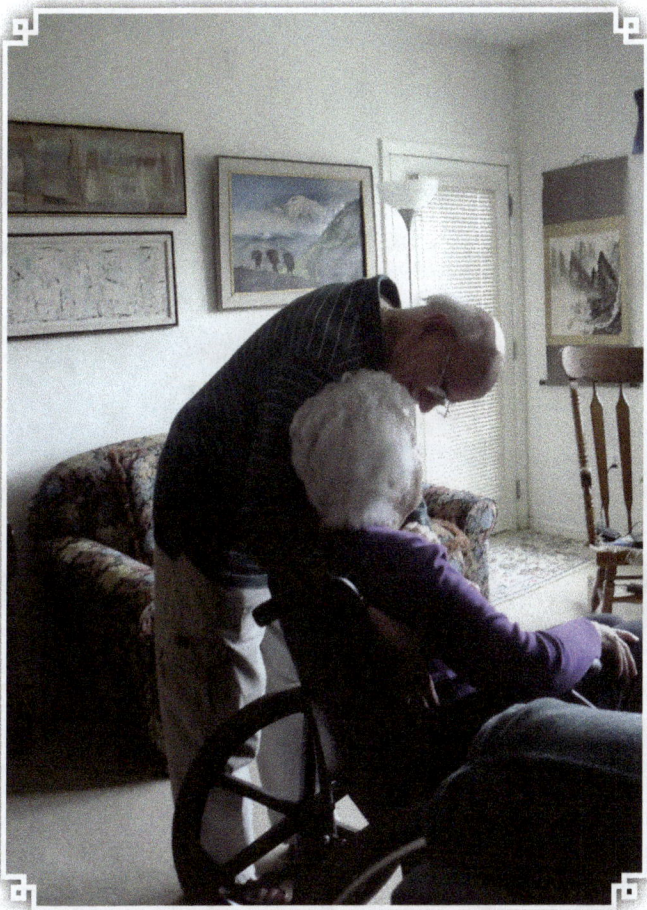

Love under the shadow, 2012

www.ingramcontent.com/pod-product-compliance
Lightning Source LLC
Chambersburg PA
CBHW050710280326
41926CB00088B/2919